Diabetes Mellitus

Its History, Chemistry, Anatomy, Pathology, Physiology, and Treatment

By William Morgan

Member of the Royal College of Surgeons, England

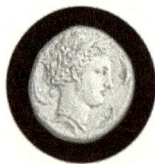

PANTIANOS
CLASSICS

Published by Pantianos Classics

ISBN-13: 978-1-78987-022-0

First published in 1877

Contents

Preface

THE following treatise has been undertaken with the view of supplying a want long needed in the field of advanced medicine — namely, a practical exposition of one of the most obscure and intractable disorders that can afflict the human body.

The scope of the work now submitted to the reader, proposes to accomplish five leading objects:

Firstly. To throw some new light on the past and present history of Diabetes Mellitus.

Secondly. To show more clearly than has hitherto been done, the frequent abnormal condition of the liver, in conjunction with a saccharine condition of the urine.

Thirdly. To review some of the most recent physiological facts connected with the subject.

Fourthly. To review some of the more obscure pathological causes of Diabetes, more particularly those which are closely allied to the centre of the nervous system.

Fifthly. To analyse the past and present treatment of the disease, in accordance with sound pathological views; and the advocacy of a purely hygienic system of auxiliaries, in accordance with the vital truths of sound physiology, to the end that the restorative energies of the organism may be placed in the best position, and have the fullest scope for their own development, thus converting diseased into healthy action: it being clearly established that the natural tendency of the body is to rectify its own abnormal conditions, when placed in the best circumstances for so doing; hence the special advocacy of Turkish Baths, Hydropathy, Gymnastics, and general Hygiene. Such was the natural, common-sense-like, and effective agency with which the illustrious SYDENHAM combated many diseases; and such, in effect, was the plan relied on by the fathers of ancient medicine — by Hippocrates, by Celsus, by Galen, Aretseus, and many more.

In conclusion, the writer may say that he has aimed at giving a perspicuous and practical exposition of the nature, causes, &c., of the complaint. He is conscious of its many imperfections, which leisure might have corrected. Such as it is, however, he ventures to submit it to the profession and an impartial public, believing that any honest and sincere attempt to correct the theory, and to improve the treatment, of a disease so largely involving human happiness as the one under discussion — a disease which has for ages baffled the skill of the faculty in all countries — will be received with a friendly feeling and liberality, and judged of with candour and unbiassed opinions.

W. M.
1, Old Steine, Brighton.
May 10th, 1877.

List of Homoeopathic Medicines Prescribed in This Work

Their Number, Official Names, Abbreviations, and the Potency Usually Prescribed by the Author

No.	Name.	Abbreviation.	English Name.	Potency.
1	Aconitum Napellus ...	Acon.	Monkshood	φ 1, 2, 3.
2	Acidum Nitricum ...	Ac. Nit. ...	Nitric Acid	1, 2, 3.
3	Acidum Hydrochloricum	Ac. Hydroch.	Hydrochloric Acid ...	1, 2, 3.
4	Acidum Phosphoricum...	Ac. Phos. ...	Phosphoric Acid ...	φ 1, 2, 3.
5	Asclepias Syriaca ...	Asc. Syr. ...	Milk-weed	φ 1, 2.
6	Alumina	Alum.... ...	Pure Clay	3, 6.
7	Ammonium Carbonicum	Ammo. C. ...	Carbonate of Ammonia.	3, 6.
8	Ambra Grisea	Amb. G. ...	Ambergris	3, 6.
9	Argentum Metallicum ...	Arg. M. ...	Silver	3, 6, 12.
10	Arnica Montana	Arn. M. ...	Leopard's Bane ...	1, 3, 6.
11	Arum Triphyllum ...	Arum Tri. ...	Cuckoo Pint ...	3, 2.
12	Arsenicum Album ...	Ars. A. ...	White Arsenic ...	2, 3.
13	Belladonna	Bell.	Deadly Nightshade ...	1, 2, 3.
14	Baryta Carbonica ...	Bar. C... ...	Carbonate of Baryta ...	2, 3, 6.
15	Calcaria Carbonica ...	Calc. C. ...	Carbonate of Lime ...	6, 12.
16	Cantharis Vesicatoria ...	Canth	Spanish Fly	2, 3, 6.
17	Carbo Vegetabilis ...	Carb. V. ...	Vegetable Charcoal ...	1, 2, 3.
18	Cinchona	Cinch.... ...	Peruvian Bark	φ 1, 2.
19	Chloral Hydrate... ...	Chl. Hyd. ...	Chloral Hydrate ...	φ 1, 2.
20	Clematis Erecta	Clem. Erect....	Upright Virgin's Bower	1, 2, 3.
21	Conium	Con.	Hemlock...	1, 2, 3.
22	Digitalis Purpurea ...	Dig.	Purple Foxglove ...	1, 2, 3.
23	Eupatorium Perfoliatum	Eup. Per. ...	Gravel Root	φ 1, 2, 3.
24	Graphites	Graph.. ...	Plumbago	6, 12.
25	Helonias Dioica	Helon.. ...	Blazing Star	φ 1, 2.
26	Kali Carbonicum ...	Kal. C... ...	Salt of Tartar	3, 6.
27	Kreasote	Kreas.... ...	Kreasote...	2, 3.
28	Lactic Acid	Lac. Ac.	Lactic Acid	φ
29	Ledum Palustre	Led. Pal. ...	Marsh Tea	φ 1, 2. : ,
30	Leptandra Virginica ...	Lep. Vir. ...	Black Root	φ 1, 2.
31	Magnesia Carbonica ...	Mag. C. ...	Carbonate of Magnesia	6.
32	Mercurius Solubilis ...	Merc. Sol. ...	Soluble Mercury ...	6.
33	Natrum Muriaticum ...	Nat. Mur. ...	Common Salt	φ 1, 2, 3.
34	Nux Vomica	Nux V. ...	Nux Vomica	1, 2, 3.
35	Plumbum Metallicum ...	Plum. M. ...	Lead	12.
36	Podophyllum Peltatum...	Podoph P. ...	May-apple	φ 1, 2.
37	Salycilic Acid	Sal. Ac. ...	Salycilic Acid	φ 1, 2.
38	Strychnine	Strych. ...	Strychnine	2, 3.
39	Sulphur	Sulph. ...	Sulphur	6.
40	Staphysagria	Staph.... ...	Staves-acre	φ 1, 3.
41	Terebinthine	Tereb.... ...	Turpentine	1, 2, 3.
42	Uranium Nitrate... ...	Uran. N. ...	Nitrate of Uranium ...	3.
43	Veratrum Album ...	Ver. A. ...	White Hellebore ...	3.

Homeopathic Medicines

*THEIR MODE OF PREPARATION; THEIR CURATIVE SELECTION; THE DOSE OR PO-
TENCY, AND THE MANNER OF THEIR ADMINISTRATION, BRIEFLY EXPLAINED.*

The Homoeopathic "Materia Medica" contains at the present time from 260 to 270 medicinal preparations; the greater number of these have been faithfully proved on man, woman, and child, while in a state of health, in order to ascertain the pathogenetic and specific properties of each drug; others have been but partially proved, and hold a place in its pages on empirical grounds.

Homoeopathic medicines are prepared and kept in the form of Tinctures, Triturations, Pilules, and Globules; a few in ether and glycerine, such as the snake poisons.

The tinctures are chiefly derived from the vegetable and animal kingdoms; known as expressed juice, mother tincture, or matrix tincture, the symbol of which is the Greek ϕ.

From these tinctures the various dilutions or potencies are prepared; and the higher we ascend in the scale of dilution the further we depart from the crude substance, which accounts for the non-poisonous, and consequently non-injurious properties of Homoeopathically prepared medicines; but they nevertheless retain medicinal properties of marvellous efficacy, which are potent against the disease; and inert against the constitution, when Homoeopathically or specifically selected. Triturations, on the contrary, are chiefly prepared from substances derived from the mineral kingdom. Among these may be enumerated sulphur, mercury, arsenic, zinc, tin, baryta, gold, silver, iron, lime, copper, alum, tellurium, and many more. The mode of preparing the various potencies from the matrix triturations is similar to those prepared from the tinctures; for the manipulation of which the reader is referred to the pages of the Homoeopathic Pharmacopoeia, recently published under the auspices of the British Homoeopathic Society.

Pilules and Globules

These little pellets, which have afforded our Allopathic brethren no scanty field for amusement and ridicule, are not in reality Homoeopathic medicines at all: they are simply elegant and ingenious little *vehicles* for the administration of the various remedies when reduced to the liquid form (tincture), and used on the same principle as Doctor Dosewell selects honey, syrup, jam, or jelly for his nauseous compound of grey powder, rhubarb, senna, or Dover's powder: — *in quovis vehiculo crasso* — in some convenient vehicle: or as once facetiously translated by a candidate for the licence of the Apothecaries' Company — in some stout hackney coach.

On the Selection of Remedies.

The fundamental principle of Homoeopathic practice — the law of cure — as discovered, demonstrated, and promulgated by Hahnemann, is simply and forcibly expressed in the following maxim: — Similia similibus curantur; which simply means that diseases are cured most quickly, safely, and effectually, by medicines which are capable of producing symptoms SIMILAR to those existing in the patient, and which characterise his disease; for in accordance with the therapeutic law of similarity, medicines cure affections similar, or like unto those they produce. The immortal bard of Avon has well expressed this law in the following lines: —

"Tut, man! one fire burns out another's burning;
   One pain is lessened by another's anguish.
Turn giddy, and be help by backward turning;
   One desperate grief cures with another's languish:
Take thou some new infection to the eye,
   And the rank poison of the old will die."

Homeopathy, then, proceeds upon the great incontrovertible truth, that as the phenomena of chemistry depend upon positive laws — as the movements and instincts of the brute creation are regulated in the most orderly manner — as the physiological functions of the human organism constitute an harmonious play of beautifully co-ordinate forces, — so nature has ordained a definite relation between *remedial* agents and *diseases.* In the discoveries of such relationship, extending over a field co-extensive with nature herself, ever fresh, ever increasing in interest, consists the study of Homoeopathy in its application as well as its practice. The treatment of disease henceforth must rest on positive and unerring laws; it cannot possibly depend on chance, but must be regulated in a manner commensurate with the unchanging principles of nature and philosophy.

While the difference of sexes in all living beings beneficently binds them together in prolific union, the crude matters of inorganic nature are impelled by like instincts. Even in the darkness of chaos, matter was accumulated or separated accordingly, as affinity or antagonistic matter attracted or repelled its various parts. The celestial fire follows the metals; the magnet, the iron; amber when rubbed attracts light bodies; earth blends with earth; salt separates from the waters of the sea and joins its like. Everything in inanimate nature hastens to associate itself with its like.

The beauteous aspect of the world, the order of the celestial bodies, the revolution of the sun, the moon, and all the stars, indicate sufficiently, at one glance, that all this is not the work of chance.

Potencies.

Homoeopathic medicines have been used by physicians at various dilutions: — from the mother tinctures to the two thousandth attenuation. For ordinary purposes, however, I would advise my readers to confine their selections from the mother tincture ϕ to the 3rd, or 6x dilution, as being the most useful and efficacious, and is moreover in accordance with the views of the majority and more advanced sections of Homoeopathic practitioners in this country and America. They constitute the ordinary potencies prescribed by the writer for many years, and have proved eminently successful in his hands.

Mode of Administration

We have observed that there are four modes of preparing the medicines: — viz., Tinctures, Triturations, medicated Pilules and Globules; there is also more than one mode of administering these remedies.

I. Tinctures. — The dose of these preparations is, as a rule, one drop administered at stated intervals.

In acute diseases, and in those severe and dangerous complaints which rapidly run their headlong course to a fatal termination — as, for instance, croup, cholera, acute atrophy of the liver, &c. — it may be necessary, at the commencement of the treatment, to repeat the dose at intervals of every ten, twenty, or thirty minutes, until a favourable impression is made on the symptoms, when the interval between the doses should be lengthened as the patient improves. For this purpose it were well to mix thoroughly twelve drops of the selected tincture in twelve table-spoonfuls of water, and administered accordingly.

In chronic diseases, there should be an interval between the repetition of the dose of from twelve to twenty-four hours; and according to the strict rules of Hahnemann, to as many days or weeks. This prolonged action of one dose of a medicine has been much doubted. I have but little faith in it myself, and generally advise that the medicine should be repeated once a day, or night and morning.

Triturations. — These preparations may be taken dry on the tongue, or in solution; one grain, or as much as will stand on the point of a penknife, is about equal to one drop of the tincture: one pilule, or six globules.

If the solution be preferred, twelve grains should be dissolved in twelve table-spoonfuls of water, well stirred, and taken according to the circumstances of the case.

Pilules and Globules. — These elegant and Liliputian medicaments may also be taken either dry on the tongue or in solution. If the former, one pilule or six globules may be considered a fair adult dose: if the latter, one pilule or six globules dissolved in a table-spoonful of water, may be considered equivalent to one drop of the tincture in the same quantity of water.

Medicines, as a rule, should be taken on an empty stomach, or about two hours after a meal.

The water used for mixing the medicine should be distilled, filtered, or cold-boiled.

The solution should be made in a clean tumbler, closely covered with half a sheet of note-paper; or in a bottle well corked and kept from dust and light.

Diet.

All articles of diet and drinks which contain medicinal properties should be strictly avoided whilst taking Homoeopathic medicines; such as coffee, green tea, and herb teas of every description; ginger, pepper, vinegar, mustard, allspice, cinnamon, and spices of all kinds; and every variety of vegetable food of an aromatic or medicinal character, as onions, garlic, radishes, celery, or parsnips; and every variety of animal food strong-scented or difficult of digestion, as old smoked meat, roof beef, bacon, fat pork, sausages, rancid butter, strong cheese, &c.

In acute diseases the diet should consist of the most light and nutritious kinds of food; such as toast-water, barley water, rice-water, panada, arrowroot gruel, and mutton broth. When the more violent symptoms of the disease have subsided, and the patient is fairly convalescent, more substantial food may be allowed in moderate quantities; such as beef-tea or chicken-tea thickened with pearl barley, arrowroot or sago, boiled rice, boiled chicken, or a sweetbread; toast, rice, and bread-pudding; and if there exists no derangement of the stomach or bowels, a few grapes, strawberries, or peaches may be taken. In chronic diseases, almost every variety of wholesome, nutritious, and easily digested food may be allowed, providing it does not answer the description of such kinds of aliments as are above prohibited.

As an ordinary beverage, pure water should be allowed in all cases, toast-water, apple-water, , barley-water, or rice-water, with an occasional glass of sound Burgundy, Carlowitz, or Somlau.

If the bowels become obstinately costive, and will not respond to the ordinary medicines prescribed in another part of this work, a recourse may be had with safety to the occasional use of saline waters — the Apollinaris, Freidrichshall, or the Hunyadi Janos of Hungary.

Introduction

THERE is no section of experimental investigations in the whole circle of medical science, that have yielded more interesting and valuable results, and that are of greater value and importance to the " Clinical Physician," than that which is allied to the study of animal saccharine matter.

Anterior to 1848, the study of "Diabetes Mellitus" was more or less in darkness and obscurity; but from that period down to the present time, an entire revolution has taken place, and a flood of light has awakened the profession from a long and dreamy slumber, and has cast a bright " halo " round our present ideas, as to a more correct and scientific knowledge of the physiology and pathology of a saccharine condition of the urine. For these valuable and important results, we are specially indebted to the searching and interesting experiments so ably conducted by Claude Bernard, Chauveau, Bruke, Bence Jones, Harley, Pavy, and others; but although much is now already known, yet much still remains to be discovered ere we are able completely to unravel the series of obscure laws which regulate the formation and destruction of saccharine matter in the animal economy. Before, however, we embark upon the consideration of the anatomy, chemistry, physiology, pathology, and therapeutics of Diabetes Mellitus, it were well to glance briefly at the early history and literature of this interesting subject, in order that we may the more clearly define and appreciate the advances which, step by step, have already been made; and to comprehend in what respect the physiological and pathological views at present advanced, differ from those of a bygone era.

While essentially intended as a popular, or semi-popular work, the different subjects are handled with strict accuracy, and according to the most recent and advanced physiological, pathological, and therapeutic views, both allopathic and in accordance with the doctrine of Hahnemann. It is consequently anticipated that this little work may not altogether be considered unworthy the attention of the profession, who may find in it some new, practical, and useful information on a subject which, till very recently, has been for ages enshrouded in so much obscurity.

Chapter One - History of Diabetes Mellitus

Definition.

THE term Diabetes — which derives its signification from the Greek word $\Delta\iota\alpha\beta\eta\tau\eta\varsigma$ a siphon; or from $\delta\iota\alpha\beta\alpha\acute{\iota}\nu\omega$, transeo; $\delta\iota\alpha$, through, and

$\beta\alpha\iota\nu\omega$, to pass — may be defined as the secretion of an inordinate quantity of sweet-tasting, violet-smelling urine; accompanied with great thirst, dryness of skin, extreme debility, and general emaciation.

Nomenclature of Diabetes Mellitus

Synonymously, Diabetes is a coinage of the two Greek words —$\delta\iota\alpha$, through, and $\beta\alpha\iota\nu\omega$, to pass. It is known as the Lienteria Urinalis of Celsus; the Tabes Urinalis of Gralen; the Diarrhoea Urinosa of Zacutus Lucitanus; the Profusio Urinse of Euych; the Dipsas of Aretseus; the Dipsacus of Paulus ginetus, the Polyuria of Seidel; the Diabetes Anglicus of Mead and Souvages; the Phthisuria Saccharina of Nicolas; the Diabetes Saccharena of Hufeland; the Diabetes Mellitus of Eollo, Cullen, and Sagar; the Dipsacus of Hecker; the Phthysuria of Eeil; the Grlucosuria of Claude Bernard.

National Nomenclature of Diabetes Mellitus

The Harnfliuss, Honigartige, Haruruhr of the Germans; the Urinflod of the Danes; the Diabete of the French; the Flosso d'ornia of the Italians; and the Urine Flux, or Saccharine Urine, of the English.

There is no particular allusion to Diabetes Mellitus to be found in the classic works of the renowned Hippocrates, the Father of Medicine, 450 B.C. Celsus and Gralen refer but slightly to it; we are, however, indebted to Aretseus the Cappadocian, and a contemporary of Galen A.D. 200; and Paulus Mgineta, particularly the former, for a very interesting and complete history of this complaint. "Diabetes," says Aretseus, "is a wonderful affection, not very frequent among men, being a melting down of the flesh and limbs into urine. The course is the common one, namely, the kidneys and bladder; for the patient never stops making water, but the flow is incessant, as if from the opening of aqueducts. The nature of the disease, then, is chronic, and it takes a long period to form; but the patient is short-lived if the constitution of the disease be completely established; for the melting is rapid, the death speedy. Moreover, life is disgusting and painful; thirst unquenchable; excessive drinking; which, however, is disproportionate to the large quantity of urine, for more urine is passed, and one cannot stop them either from drinking or making water. Or if for a time they abstain from drinking, their mouth becomes parched, and their body dry; the viscera seem as if scorched up; they are affected with nausea, restlessness, and a burning thirst; and at no distant term they expire. Thirst, as if scorched up with fire. But by what method could they be restrained from making water? Or how can shame become more potent than pain? And even if they were to restrain themselves for a short time, they become swelled in the loins, scrotum, and hips; and when they give vent, they discharge the collected urine, and the swellings subside, for the oversow passes to the bladder.

"If the disease be fully established, it is strongly marked; but if it be merely coming on, the patients have the mouth parched, saliva white, frothy, as from thirst (for the thirst is not yet confirmed), weight in the hypochondriac region. A sensation of heat, or of cold from the stomach to the bladder is, as it were, the advent of the approaching disease; they now make a little more water than usual, and there is thirst, but not yet great.

"But if it increase still more, the heat is small indeed, but pungent, and seated in the intestines; the abdomen is shrivelled, the veins protuberant, general emaciation, when the quantity of urine and thirst have already increased; and when, at the same time, the sensation appears at the extremity of the member, the patients immediately make water. Hence the disease appears to me to have got the name of DIABETES, as if from the Greek word διαβαίνω (which signifies a siphon), because the fluid does not remain in the body, but uses the man's body as a ladder whereby to leave it. They stand out for a certain time, though not very long, for they pass urine with pain, and the emaciation is dreadful; nor does any great portion of the drink get into the system, and many parts of the flesh pass out along with the urine."

CAUSES. — "The cause of Diabetes," says the same illustrious author, "may be, that some one of the acute diseases may have terminated in this; and during the crisis, the disease may have left some malignity lurking in the part. It is not improbable, also, that something pernicious, derived from other diseases which attack the bladder and kidneys, may sometimes prove the cause of this affection. But if any one is bitten by the Dipsas, [1] the affection induced by the wound is of this nature; for the reptile— the Dipsas — if it bite one, kindles up an unquenchable thirst. For they drink copiously, not as a remedy for the thirst, but so as to produce repletion of the bowels by the insatiable desire of drink. But if one be pained by the thirst and distension of the bowels, and feels uncomfortable, and abstains from drink for a little, he again drinks copiously from thirst, and thus the evil alternates; for the thirst and the drink alternate together. Others do not pass urine, nor is there any relief from what is drank. Wherefore, what from insatiable thirst, or overflow of liquids, and distension of the belly, the patients have suddenly burst."

Those celebrated Greek commentators, Oribasius, Aetius, Alexander of Tralles, and Paulus Aegineta, who represented the medicine of ancient Greece during that eventful period of transition which comruenced at the death of Gralen, the great Roman physician, A.D. 200, to the 14th and 15th century, refer to Diabetes in clear and unmistakable terms; but they added nothing, either to the pathology or treatment of the complaint, beyond drawing a comparison between it and Lientery, [2] and that the one affection differs from the other, in as far as, that the undigested aliments pass off — in the former by the urine, in the latter by the stools; — an opinion which was afterwards embraced by John Fern el, Duret, Zacutus Lucitanus and others, all able representatives of the Erudite School of that period. All these physicians gave to the disease the name of Diabetes, a term derived from the Greek $\delta\iota\alpha$, through; and $\beta\alpha\iota\nu\omega$, I go.

Paulus Aegineta describes Diabetes "as a rapid passage of the drink out of the body, liquids being voided by urine as they were drank; and hence it is attended with immoderate thirst; and therefore the affection has been called Dipsacus, being occasioned by a weakness of the retentive faculty of the kidneys, while the attractive is increased in strength, and deprives the whole body of its moisture by its immoderate heat. Wherefore with this intention we will give more food, and that of difficult digestion, and not hurried, such as alica with rose-wine, or rhodomel, hydromel, or some wine that is not old, or some of the hot wines. We must give of pot-herbs, succory, endive, and lettuces; of fishes, those that abide among rocks; the feet and womb of swine; pears, apples, and pomegranates; and give cold water to drink. They must get to drink propomata, [3] from the juice of knot-grass, and elicampane, in dark-coloured wine, and from the decoction of dates, and myrtles. We must apply a cataplasm to the hypochondrium and kidneys of polenta, in vinegar and rose-oil; and of the leaves of the vine and navelwort, pellitory of the wall, and purslain. We must promote sweats, and excite vomiting by drinking cold water; and make them abstain from all sorts of diuretics. There will be nothing improper in letting blood at the commencement."

Such is a brief outline of the views taken by those ancient physicians relative to Diabetes and its treatment, at a period which may be estimated as the 2nd century of the Christian era.

It was not, however, till 1674 that a rational theory of Diabetes Mellitus was first advanced; and that the urine voided possessed A SWEET TASTE: the honour of which discovery belongs to one of England's pioneers in the field of medical science — by name Thomas Willis, and a prominent member of the ItroChemical School of Medicine during the reformed era. From this time henceforth, the disease was divided into two distinct types: 1. Diabetes Insipidus, or that which had no sugar. 2. Diabetes Mellitus, or that which had sugar. From that time also, down to the present day, opinions as to its physiology and pathology have been various; and the remedies recommended for its cure still more diversified. Even down to the present time the term Diabetes has been applied to various conditions of disease: namely, to that consisting chiefly of diuresis — which is a morbidly-increased flow of urine, without any reference to its chemical constituents; — to that in which the urine is voided, not only more frequently, and in larger quantity than natural, but also of changed quality, as regard certain of its abnormal constituents; namely, urea, and uric-acid, and albumen, &c.; — and lastly, to that in which saccharine matter is either super-added to the other ingredients contained in the urine, or in part replaces them. It is to the last of these abnormal conditions of the urine that I shall limit the term Diabetes, and which is conformable with the views of most pathologists. By tracing the history of Diabetes Mellitus a little further on, we shall find, that in 1774, just a century after

Willis's discovery, another important secret was brought to light by one Matthew Dobson of Liverpool; who discovered that the blood, as well as the urine, in Diabetes Mellitus, contained sugar; and from this fact he very rightly came to the conclusion, that the saccharine matter found in the urine was not manufactured in, but only excreted by, the kidneys.

In 1778 — just four years afterwards — another Englishman, by name Cowley, succeeded in separating the saccharine matter from the urine in a free state.

In 1796, Dr. J. Rollo, a surgeon in the Royal Artillery, made the first important observation relative to the treatment of Diabetes Mellitus, by discovering that animal diet not only reduces the quantity of urine, but that it also diminishes the amount of saccharine matter daily eliminated.

In 1815, M. Chevreul, a French physician, ascertained that the saccharine matter found in Diabetic urine, differs from ordinary CANE sugar; and that it closely resembles that of the GRAPE.

In 1825, Tiedmann and Gmelin gained another important step, by discovering that starchy matter is transformed into sugar during its passage along the intestinal canal.

In 1837, the next observation of interest was made by a Scotch physician, by name McGregor, of Glasgow; who discovered saccharine matter in the vomited matter of Diabetic patients. From this fact he was induced to attribute Diabetes to faulty digestion. A similar view was taken by the late Dr. Proiit; for in his able work on " Stomach and Renal Diseases," 5th edition, p. 38, he says, " The facts and observations I have to offer on the subject are founded on the opinion already advanced; namely — that Diabetes is nothing more nor less than a form of Dyspepsia; that this Dyspepsia principally consists in a difficulty of assimilating the saccharine alimentary principle; and like all other forms of Dyspepsia, whether it be an inherited or an induced affection. Diabetes is liable to be much modified and aggravated by concomitant circumstances." Eollo also, at the close of the 18th century, set forth a similar opinion, that Diabetes Mellitus was chiefly due to imperfect digestion — to a derangement having its seat in the stomach, and attributable to a peculiar alteration in the "gastric juice," which had acquired the alleged morbid property of changing into sugar the vegetable materials ingested.

This theory, however, was completely exploded by the observations and experimental investigations of Tiedmann and Grmelin, who ascertained, that during the process of digestion of starchy substances, sugar is produced as a natural phenomenon. Magendie also further ascertained, that, during the process of digestion of amylaceous matter, the blood in the portal system is charged with sugar. From this it followed, that the formation of sugar in the digestive canal, from vegetable materials, could be no longer legitimately looked upon as forming the source of the saccharine matter in Diabetes, because such an event had been clearly shown to take place as a natural sequence to the process of digestion. If we pursue our historical investigation

but one step further, we shall encounter an entirely new phase in the literature and position of Diabetes Mellitus, in which we shall find, that the clinical
teachings of the sick chamber have given way to those of the laboratory.

It is now over twenty-eight years ago — 1848 — since that eminent experimental physiologist, Claude Bernard, after a series of scientific investigations, proclaimed to the astonished world, that animals, as well as vegetables,
possessed a sugar-creating function. Until these investigations brought to
light this startling and remarkable phenomena, all the saccharine matter
found in the human body, whether in its normal or abnormal condition, was
supposed to spring from the transformation of vegetable matter alone; and
now for the first time were we. cognizant of the astounding fact, that the
HUMAN RACE, like sugarcanes, possess a sugar-manufacturing organ — the
liver. In fact, that marvellous gland is as busily and actively engaged, both
hourly and daily, in fabricating sugar, as it is in manufacturing and secreting
bile.

Like all great discoveries, the rays it shadows forth are broadly reflected
over the varied departments of scientific medicine: by it new and enlight-
ened ideas have been brought to light, and within the grasp of man: by it new
and important discoveries have been made, both in the dead-house, the laboratory, the clinical ward, and in the sick chamber.

In 1849, Claude Bernard made another and most important discovery; —
he proved that Diabetes Mellitus can be artificially induced in animals by
pricking the floor of the fourth ventricle of the brain.

In 1851, Dr. George Harley ascertained, that Diabetes Mellitus can be artificially induced in animals by means of stimulants, introduced directly into
the portal circulation in the form of alcohol. This clearly explains why Diabetes is to be found much more frequently in spirit-drinking than in other
countries.

In 1855, Claude Bernard further discovered, that the formation of sugar in
the liver cannot be regarded in the light of a " vital process" — as it goes on,
not only after the death of the animal, but even after the removal of the organ
from the body.

In 1865 — 67, George Harley and M. Chauveau conjointly ascertained, that
the sugar normally present in the circulation is not burned off in the lungs, as
formerly believed by most physiologists; but that it disappears from the
blood in its transit through the minute blood-vessels (capillaries) of the general circulation, from whence it most probably goes to nourish the body.

In 1857, Claude Bernard is again digging up fresh treasures in the same
field; and finds that, before albuminous substances are converted into saccharine matter, they first pass through the transitional stage of Glucogene —
animal starch.

In 1859-60 Bruke ascertained, by a series of careful and minute investigations, that traces of sugar are found in normal urine. This has since been confirmed by Dr. Bence Jones, in 1865. Harley regards this discovery as a fun-

damental law: that in diseases, neither new substances nor new functions are created; morbid phenomena being merely the result of a change in the quantity and quality of normally existing agents and agencies. Finally, in 1872, M.M. Cyon and Aladoff related, before the Academy of Sciences of St. Petersburg, some interesting experiments they had undertaken to elucidate the origin of Diabetes Mellitus. It was found, that irritation of the fibres of the annulus of Vieussens, [4] produced white marks on the lobules of the liver, which appeared on the cessation of the irritation. These were in the position of the branches of the portal vein and hepatic artery, to the contraction of one or both of which they were believed to be due; and other experiments seemed to point to the artery.

It is concluded that the vaso-motor nerves of the artery are within the annulus of Vieussens. Their division causes the artery to dilate, and, at the same time, gives rise to a saccharine condition of the urine.

[1] The Dipsas was a species of viper, also referred to by Galen, Avicenna, and Paul Aegineta.
[2] A species of diarrhoea, in which the food has been only partially digested.
[3] Propomata; a beverage made of strong wine and aromatic herbs.
[4] Raymond Vieussens, a great discoverer in the anatomy of the brain and nervous system. Lyons, 1685.

Chapter Two - The Anatomy of Diabetes Mellitus

MORBID anatomy has contributed but little towards elucidating the pathology of Diabetes Mellitus in very many cases. We too often refer the origin of the saccharine matter, encountered in this malady, to an abnormal action of the liver; but no special structural change has hitherto been discovered in this gland, such as we find, for instance, in the kidney, under the existence of Albuminuria; in the supra-renal capsules, under the existence of the bronzed skin of Addison; in the right side of the heart, under the existence of hypertrophy, chronic inflammation, fatty or waxy degeneration of the liver; in the trachea, under the existence of croup; and in the valves of the heart and the cylo-poetic vessels, under the existence of dropsical effusions. We have here, and in many other cases, simply an outward manifestation of a disordered functional action to deal with, in the absence of any prominent anatomical lesion to account for it. Diabetes Mellitus, in this respect, bears a strong analogy to Jaundice, Ascites, and Anasarca; being simply symptoms, outward manifestations, or symptomatic landmarks, as it were, of some grave internal disorder. It is, in fact, the supplicating voice of Nature, appealing to the physician for help and relief. The only abnormality hitherto found in a Diabetic liver, consists of the organ being darker in colour; firm and tough in consistence; larger in size, and uniform in contour. The bile is often found thick and turbid, and of a red or brownish-red colour. On standing, there is thrown down a copious sediment, which, when microscopically examined, has been found to consist of yellow, amorphous, or granular-looking matter, with columnar-shaped epithelial cells.

There are, however, various morbid appearances to be met with in divers organs of the body, which are allied, or supposed to be allied, to a saccharine condition of the urine; but many of those only constitute effects, and do not therefore essentially belong to, or primarily cause, the disease. Disease of the lungs, for instance, forms a no uncommon concomitant of Diabetes Mellitus. It generally assumes a simple inflammatory form, with a deposit of little masses of grey hepatized lung — the "Pneumonic Phthisis" of Addison. The proneness, in Diabetes Mellitus, to its invasion, may be regarded as dependent upon the morbid condition which the blood has acquired by virtue of the presence of saccharine matter: remove this, and the susceptibility in question no longer exists. Many pathologists view this condition of the lungs as true Tuberculosis: but the extensive experience of Dr. Wilks, in the anatomical theatre of Guy's Hospital, clearly proves that the condition referred to, results from simple inflammation, and is doubtless caused by the irritating particles of sugar constantly passing through the delicate structure of the lungs — although it may terminate in a breakdown of the lung-tissue, and terminate in the formation of cavities.

Recent investigations, however, go far to prove, that we are at last on the high road to a more correct diagnosis as to the CAUSES of Diabetes Mellitus, the origin of which has so long been hidden in darkness and obscurity, and which shall receive due consideration when we come to discuss the pathology of this no less intricate and interesting subject.

Chapter Three - Physical and Chemical Properties of Healthy Urine

THE normal properties of healthy urine, recently ' voided, have the temperatures of the body. The excretion is transparent and of a light amber colour. Its odour is peculiar; but not unpleasant; its taste is salt, and bitter. On cooling its peculiar odour disappears; and its specific gravity ranges from 1.005 to 1.033.

CHEMICALLY — healthy urine has a slight ACID reaction. It remains unchanged when heated to the boiling point; nor does it yield any precipitate with mineral acids.

Oxalic Acid produces a slight cloud of oxalate of lime.

Free Alkalies throw down a phosphate of lime.

The Salts of Baryta, silver, and lead, cause precipitates.

Tannin, slight cloudiness.

Healthy Urine holds in solution, water, urea, uric acid, lactic acid, carbonic, hydrochloric, sulphuric, and phosphoric acids; in combination with the bases of soda, potash, ammonia, magnesia, and lime; with vesical mucus, and extractive matters; hippuric acid, and, according to the investigations of Bruke and Bence Jones, slight traces of sugar.

The quantity of healthy urine voided in the twenty-four hours, varies considerably in different persons; and in the same persons at different times of the day; and at different seasons.

Haller calculated the quantity at forty-nine ounces.

Keil at thirty-eight ounces.

Prout at thirty-two ounces — 30 oz. in summer and 40 oz. in winter.

Christison at thirty-five ounces.

Raeyer from twenty-one to fifty-seven ounces.

Simon about forty-five ounces.

Dalton about forty-eight and a-half ounces in November, and fifty-one and a-half in the month of June.

The average estimate of these experiments is about forty-one ounces, or a little more than two imperial pints; and the urine amounts to more than half the entire solid and liquid ingesta.

The density, also, of healthy urine varies; and ranges from 1.010 to 1.031.

It is denser in males than it is in females: it increases from childhood to manhood, and falls again in old age; it is increased by hot weather; by much exercise; by free perspiration; by a very dry diet; by animal diet; by substances containing much azote; by the meal of dinner; and during sleep.

It is diminished by cold; by sedentary habits; by a water-diet; by vegetable food; by acids; and by alcoholic fluids.

Chapter Four - Physical and Chemical Properties of Diabetic Urine

DIABETES MELLITUS is one of those forms of disease which demands for its careful -' diagnosis the science of chemistry, and some of the appliances of the laboratory. It is, however, to be observed, that the experienced physician may, from the general history of the case, pretty safely surmise the existence of the malady; but to be positive upon the point an analysis of the urine becomes an absolute necessity; although, in the generality of cases, the use of the ukinometer is all that is required.

In submitting the urine to a careful analysis, there are two important points to be gained.

The first is, to ascertain whether there exists any saccharine matter or not?

The second is — in the event of sugar being found — to determine the quantity that is being passed in a given time — say twenty-four hours; as the effect of any mode of treatment can only with precision be watched by a series of quantitative examinations of the urine being conducted from time to time, and at stated hours of the day.

Chemists have drawn broad distinctions between the different forms of saccharine matters, the properties of which vary considerably; but for our present purpose I shall divide them into the two following forms.

1. That which constitutes CANE SUGAR.
2. That which constitutes GRAPE SUGAR.

A. CANE SUGAR. is a sweet principle, and very (generally diffused throughout the vegetable kingdom. In the East and West Indies, South America, the Canaries and Australia, it is chiefly obtained from the sugar-cane.

In Indo-China, and some parts of India, from certain kinds of palms.

In France and Germany, also in Norfolk, from the beet-root.

In America, from the maple. It is also found in many fruits and roots.

Sugar-cane, when allowed to crystallise slowly from its solution, forms large crystals of hydrated sugar — the "sugar-candy" of commerce, and forms oblique rhombic prisms. Sugar combines with alkalies, and after a time the alkaline reaction disappears, and an acid (the glucic) is formed.

B. GRAPE SUGAR, when crystallised, forms the sugar of fruits, or glucose: it is found in the grape, and in other fruits, and differs in many particulars from cane sugar, besides, in containing more oxygen and hydrogen. It is less sweet, less soluble in water, and crystallises in warty granular masses, and combines, with difficulty, with lime, baryta, and oxide of lead. Its solution becomes brown when heated with caustic potash, which does not calour cane sugar. It dissolves in sulphuric acid without blackening. On the contrary, Sulphuric acid chars cane sugar, and when boiled with dilute sulphuric acid, it is converted into grape sugar.

Experimentally — These changes may be simply illustrated thus. Boil a little " sugar-candy" — a sugar which we shall designate as of the first class — with potash, no apparent change will be visible; whereas, if before boiling with the potash, we heat the solution of sugar-candy in a test-tube, along with a couple of drops of hydrochloric acid, and on adding the potash, the whole liquid becomes of a dark-brown colour, in consequence of the grape sugar, which we will designate as a second-class product, which was formed by the action of the hydrochloric acid upon the cane sugar, being instantly decomposed by the potash into the acids of molasses — glucic and melassic acid.

Just as the vegetable kingdom furnishes us with the two great types of sugar — the CANE and the GRAPE — so the animal kingdom yields to us their analogues, in the form of MILK (the saccharum lactis) and LIVER sugar, or Glucogene of Claude Bernard: Milk sugar being the analogue of cane; and the liver sugar that of the grape. In further illustration of this, the sugar of milk is readily crystallised; is unaffected by alkalies; but is easily transformed into liver sugar (Glucogene) by acids. Liver sugar, on the other hand, is with difficulty crystallised; it is unaffected by acids, but is rapidly decomposed by alkalies. From experiments made by Berthelot and De Luca, it was found that, by combining liver sugar with common salt, large colourless transparent crystals were obtained, the watery solution of which ferments with yeast, and reduces the oxide of copper. From this we are led to conclude, that liver sugar, or Glucogene, is not only exactly the same as that found in Diabetic urine, but that it is also identical with the sugar of the grape. Moreover, the relative distribution of the two classes of sugar in the vegetable and animal kingdom, is nearly identical; for just as, in the vegetable world, the sugars of the SECOND CLASS greatly preponderate over those of the FIRST — so, in the animal economy, while the second-class sugar is to be encountered in the blood, the liver, and in the urine, that of the first class is limited to *mammary* secretion alone.

Tests, and Other Appliances for The Detection and Analysis of Saccharine Urine

The tools which are deemed essential for the detection and analysis, both quantitatively and otherwise, of sugar in the urine consists of —
1. A pair of well balanced weighing scales.
2. Urinometer.
3. Graduated glass measures.
4. Test-tubes.
5. A spirit lamp.
6. Density beads, or bulbs.
7. A picknometer.
8. Fermentation test-tube.
9. Litmus paper. Red and blue.
10. A two-ounce, well-grounded glass-stoppered bottle, to hold liquor-potassae; ditto, to hold a solution of sulphate of copper; ditto, to hold a solution of cupro-potassium.

For ordinary cases, or when we wish to test the urine at the bedside of the patient, a urinometer, test-tube, a little liquor-potassse and a lighted candle will generally suffice; but when we wish to be considered learned, as well as scientific, we should go through a more intricate and elaborate process.

How to Detect Sugar, and Separate That Abnormal Product from The Urine.

There are various tests in vogue for the detection of saccharine matter in the urine, which I shall now briefly dwell upon: some are simple; the others are complicated, unsatisfactory, and uncertain.

1. The presence of sugar in the urine may, for instance, sometimes be detected by the taste, particularly if we first evaporate the urine to the consistence of a syrup; but this test is not only unpleasant to the taste and imagination, but. it is also inconvenient in daily practice, and not to be relied upon.

2. When the suspected urine voided, exceeds in volume four pints in the course of the day, and yields, by that handy little instrument, the urinometer, a specific gravity exceeding 1.030, and is at the same time of a pale straw-colour, transparent, and devoid of any deposit on cooling, it may, as a rule, be taken for granted that it holds in solution saccharine matter. And when the daily quantity passed is much larger, and yields a still higher specific gravity — which the urinometer will faithfully tell us — then there can be no doubt whatever in the matter.

URINOME-TER.

Test-tube.

It must, however, be borne in mind, that the urine may contain traces of sugar even when its specific gravity is down to 1.015 or 1.012, or indeed even below its normal standard: for the delicate researches of Bruke, which were afterwards fully confirmed by the late Dr. Bence Jones, and others prove that traces of saccharine matter is present in the normal urine.

Density Beads.

The specific gravity of Diabetic urine, ranges from 1.020 to 1.050, or even 60. Hence when the symptoms lead us to suspect the presence of saccharine matter, one of the following tests should be applied for its detection. The first is undoubtedly the urinometer, and a most convenient and valuable little instrument it is, — consisting of a blown glass float, a small oblong bulb weighted with mercury, and a graduated stem ranging from 10 to 60, like A. All that is required with this instrument is, to pop it into B, a large size footed test-tube, [1] winch contains the urine, and read off the number which happens to be on a level with the surface of the liquid. If it chance to be at 15 B, then the urine has a specific gravity of 1.015. If, on the other hand, the instrument is high in the liquid, and the reading is at 30 or 40, the urine is proportionately heavy, containing, in fact, a palpable amount of sugar, its density being 1.030 or 1.040.

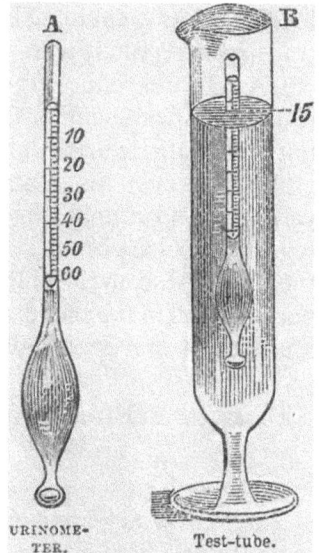

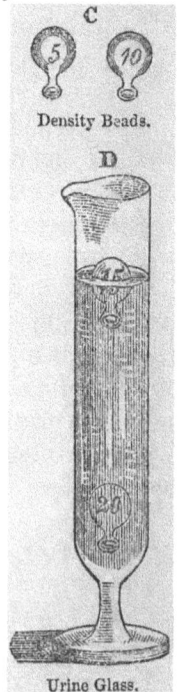

Urine Glass.

A second mode of ascertaining the specific gravity of saccharine urine is by means of DENSITY BEADS or bulbs; they are made of glass, and present the form shown in the accompanying sketch, letter C, and such as were formerly used in ascertaining the specific gravity of spirit.

These beads are numbered 5, 10, 15, 25, &c., and are gradually dropped into the urine until one sinks to the bottom of the vessel, when by reading off the number on the last bead that floated, the specific gravity of the liquid is ascertained. In the urine glass it will bp observed, that bead 20 being too heavy, has sunk to the bottom, while bead 15 is floating at the top. The specific gravity of the liquid is therefore 1.015. There are various objections, however, to this mode of testing, and it is but seldom used.

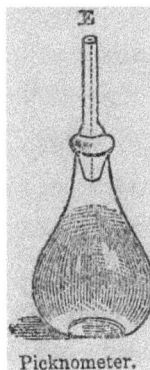

A third mode is by the use of a little instrument called the Picknometer, which is shown in the woodcut E. It is a small bottle, with a long stopper perforated by a capillary tube.

Picknometer.

When the stopper is urine Glass, accurately adjusted, the bottle holds exactly 20 ounces of distilled water. To ascertain the specific gravity of the urine by its means, the bottle is filled to overflowing, accurately stoppered, wiped dry, and weighed; and the difference between its weight, when filled with distilled water, and with urine, indicates the specific gravity. This process, however, is not often adopted for ordinary purposes.

A fourth mode of ascertaining the presence and quantity of sugar in the urine, is that known as the Fermentation test. This test was first suggested by Professor Christison: and usually known as Christison's test. The apparatus, suggested by Harley and Pavy, is simple enough as delineated in the following woodcut, F, p. 28. It consists of an ordinary test-tube, to which a tightly fitting cork is adapted, through which a piece of bent glass-tubing passes, as presented in the sketch. The urine to be picknometer. examined is mixed with a moderate quantity of ordinary yeast, or dry German yeast first mixed with a little water, and poured into the test-tube until it is completely filled. The cork is then applied, and forced into its place, taking particular care that no air is allowed to remain within the test-tube. As represented in the drawing, one limb of the piece of bent tubing passes through the test-tube until it very nearly touches the bottom. The apparatus, thus arranged, is now to be immersed in a vessel of tepid water, of a temperature not below 70° Fahrenheit. Should the urine be saccharine, minute air bubbles will speedily make their appearance, and in the course of aa hour or so a very definite quantity of carbonic acid gas is produced,

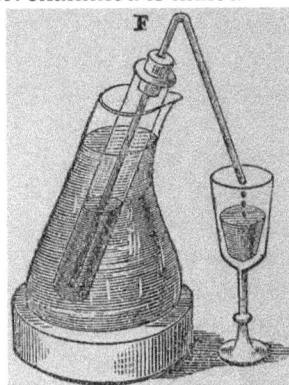

The vessel for holding the tepid water, in which is immersed the test-tube.

and. rising to the top, drives out the liquid through the bent glass into a vessel placed for its reception.

It is a well-known property of sugar — the one it enjoys — of undergoing conversion into alcohol and carbonic acid gas when brought into contact with yeast, and exposed to moderate warmth. Both grape and cane sugar are susceptible of this change, but the former is found to be more freely so than the latter. Indeed, it is thought that cane sugar has to be converted by the ferment into grape sugar before it undergoes fermentation; and the agent endowed with the power of producing this change, consists of living cells, constituting a low form of vegetable growth, which has received the name of Torula Cerevisiae.

The quantity of sugar in the urine may be readily determined, with a fair approach to accuracy, by the fermentation test, by using another apparatus as suggested by Christison: every cubic inch of carbonic acid gas given off by fermentation, corresponds in round numbers with one grain of sugar; or forty-seven of gas to forty-five of sugar. Hence the quantity of sugar may be easily found by filling a graduated tube with mercury, leaving space for a little more than the requisite quantity of urine, which is then to be introduced; next filling up what remains of the space with yeast, and, with the finger on the open end of the tube, reversing the tube in a vessel of mercury, and then placing the apparatus where it may be exposed to a heat of 70 degrees Fahrenheit for twelve to twenty-four hours.

The purely chemical tests for the detection of sugar, are those which are generally known as —

1. Moore's 'test, with liquor-potassae. Directions. Pour a small quantity of the suspected urine — say, a dessert spoonful into a test-tube; add to it about half its bulk of liquor-potassae; hold it over the flame of a spirit lamp for one or more minutes, till it boils; when the urine will assume an orange brown colour, of a depth proportionate to the quantity of sugar. This change is caused by the formation of glucic acid, which becomes transformed into melassic acid. The intensity of colour produced depends on the quantity of sugar present, which varies from a pale sherry, to a port wine, or Burgundy.

2. Trommer's test, with a solution of sulphate of copper, and liquor-potassae. Directions. Pour about a dessert spoonful of the suspected urine into a test tube; add to it a few drops of the copper solution, so as to produce a pale blue colour; then add liquor potassae in excess, until the hydrated oxide of copper first thrown down is re-dissolved, as it always is, when sugar is present, and a clear deep blue fluid is produced; boil the liquid over a spirit lamp, and if the quantity of sugar is minute, a yellowish-red opalescent tint will be produced; but if the quantity of sugar is large, then a quantity of orange-coloured precipitate — the sub-oxide of copper — is thrown down. If, however, no sugar be present, boiling the urine yields a dark-green precipitate.

These two tests, for the detection of Diabetic sugar, are considered quite sufficient for ordinary clinical examinations, although there are others which are still more delicate, viz. —

3. Runge's test, with dilute sulphuric acid. Directions. Evaporate a small quantity of the suspected urine on a surface of white porcelain, or watch-glass — say one half, or a teaspoonful; add to the warm liquid a few drops of dilute sulphuric acid, of the following strength — one part of acid to six of water. If sugar be present, the evaporated substance becomes of a deep-brown or black colour, from its conversion into carbon. This test, however delicate, must be used with caution, for albumen yields similar results.

4. Fehling's test, with cupro-potassium. This is often substituted for Trommer's; indeed, Pavy has seldom used any other for many years past; and gives the following formula, for its preparation:—

Sulphate of copper	320 grains.
Tartrate of potash (neutral)	640 "
Caustic potash (potassa fusa)	1280 "
Distilled water	20 fluid ounces.

In making the solution, the sulphate of copper is dissolved in 10 ounces of the water, and the tartrate of potash and caustic potash together in the remainder. The solution of copper is then poured into that of the tartrate and caustic potash; the combined liquid thus obtained is clear and bright, and of a beautiful deep blue colour. This solution is capable of being employed for estimating the amount, as well as for detecting the presence, of sugar.

Sugar, however, is not the only organic principle by which the copper test is reduced; as it is stated that tannin, glycerine, cellulose, leucine, uric acid, and chloroform, are capable of exerting more or less reducing action upon it. The copper test is a very delicate one, and will display the presence of minute quantities of sugar in the urine without any preliminary preparation. When, however, an exceedingly minute quantity is being looked for, the urine should be concentrated by evaporation, and treated with an excess of acetate of lead to get rid of colouring and other solid matters in the form of precipitate. The lead contained in the filtrate, belonging to the excess of acetate employed, is best removed by a stream of sulphurated hydrogen; and after a second filtration, the copper test may be applied.

Dr. Bence Jones, in a very able paper which appeared in the " Quarterly Journal of the Chemical Society," April, 1861, gives an analysis of the relative merits of different processes for the detection of minute quantities of sugar in the urine.

By means of these processes, as recommended by Bruke, the seventh part of a grain of grape sugar, dissolved in about seven fluid ounces of urine, is not only to be detected, but two-thirds of it may be actually recovered.

Dr. Henry has given us a very useful table, showing the quantity of solid extract in a wine pint of urine of different specific gravities from 1.020 to 1.050. The following abstract of this table will enable the reader to ascertain the quantity of solid matter Diabetic urine may contain.

The table enables us to ascertain with considerable precision the quantity of solid matter voided by a Diabetic patient in a given time. Thus, suppose 10 pints are passed in 24 hours, of the average specific gravity 1.040, it is evident that this will contain 10 X 1..4..2..6 = 15..7..2, or upwards of a pound and a quarter of solid extract.

Specific gravity compared with 1000 parts of water at 60°.	Quantity of solid extract in a wine pint.	Quantity of solid extract in a wine pint.			
	Grains.	oz.	dr.	scr.	grs.
1020	382.4	0	6	1	2
1021	401.6	0	6	2	1
1022	420.8	0	7	0	0
1023	440.0	0	7	1	0
1024	459.2	0	7	1	19
1025	478.4	0	7	2	18
1026	497.6	1	0	0	17
1027	516.8	1	0	1	16
1028	536.0	1	0	2	16
1029	555.2	1	1	0	15
1030	574.4	1	1	1	14
1031	593.6	1	1	2	13
1032	612.8	1	2	0	12
1033	632.0	1	2	1	12
1034	651.2	1	2	2	11
1035	670.4	1	3	0	10
1036	689.6	1	3	1	9
1037	708.8	1	3	2	8
1038	728.0	1	4	0	8
1039	747.2	1	4	1	7
1040	766.4	1	4	2	6
1041	785.6	1	5	0	5
1042	804.8	1	5	1	4
1043	824.0	1	5	2	3
1044	843.2	1	6	0	3
1045	862.4	1	6	1	2
1046	881.6	1	6	2	1
1047	900.8	1	7	0	0
1048	920.0	1	7	1	0
1049	939.2	1	7	1	19
1050	958.4	1	7	2	18

[1] Any glass vessel of sufficient depth will answer the purpose quite as well.

Chapter Five - The Symptoms of Diabetes

ON a careful examination of the clinical history of Diabetes Mellitus, from its incipient stage to its fatal termination, we are able to point out, that its progress is capable of being divided into two distinct stages, each having its special characteristics and well-marked symptoms.

Dr. Jaccoud of Paris, in a very able monograph on this complaint, points out that its primitive or fundamental symptoms — those which he considers to be essential to the disease — are five in number; namely —

1. A saccharine impregnation of the urine, known as Glycosuria, or Melituria.

2. An excess of the urinary secretion, or Polyuria.

3. An excess of thirst, known as Poly-dipsia.

4. An inordinate appetite, or Poly-phagia.

5. General emaciation, known as Auto-phagia.

The first four of these symptoms he considers to be concomitant in their origin, but the fifth he sets down for a later period, and marks the transitional stage — the commencement of wasting, or general cachexia.

The symptoms of the first stage of the disease develop themselves secretly and insidiously; and it is but seldom that either the patient or doctor is able to point out the exact period of its commencement; although Prout has stated, that in several instances he has been able to trace attacks very nearly to their origin, by ascertaining the time when the urine WAS LAST OBSERVED TO BE TURBID — an index worth remembering. The earliest symptoms known, by which the development of Diabetes may be recognised, may be set down as follows: —

A patient so afflicted, complains of an indefinable general indisposition, with debility, or prostration of muscular power as well as nervous energy; he feels fatigued or even exhausted after moderate exertion, and complains of listlessness, and disinclination for either bodily or mental exertion. He remains in bed longer than usual, is disinclined to rise, and his friends, " in their ignorance," are kindly disposed to call him lazy and that he shirks his daily task. He complains of numbness and loss of sensation over the outer and anterior surface of the thighs; and of a dull aching pain in the loins, which is of frequent occurrence. He complains of dimness of vision, and an inability to read; and occasionally there is dyspepsia, for which the disease is, at this period, often mistaken. At this early development of the disease, there is not as a rule much THIRST, but the mouth feels CLAMMY and frothy, more especially during conversation. The skin is not at this stage particularly dry, neither is the urine particularly increased in quantity, which ranges from three to six pints in the twenty-four hours, and is of a pale straw colour, transparent, and does not throw down any deposit on cooling. Dr. Prout observes, as the result of his extensive experience, that during the early stage of the disease, as a general rule, the increased flow of urine was not so great as to attract the special attention of his patients for some weeks, and in some instances for even several months, after its saccharine condition had most probably become fully established. The odour from Diabetic urine is peculiar, and " pathognomonic " of the complaint. By Guy it has been compared to that of new-made hay; by Copland to sweet whey, or milk, or violets; by Pavy to an acid smell, which he thinks is due to the occurrence of the lactic acid fermentation; it is not, says that author, unlike the smell perceived where ripe apples are stored.

The duration of the first stage is very indefinite, and varies considerably according to a variety of circumstances; it may extend over many months; and, as a rule, it is of shorter duration in youth than it is in manhood, the middle, or the more advanced period of life.

SECOND STAGE.— The symptoms which characterise the second stage become gradually superadded and blended as it were with the first, and are more or less generated out of the greater intensity acquired by the disease: and not only do we now observe the development of new symptoms, but those already existing assume a graver and more important character. Consequently, the debility of the patient, the loss of nervous energy, and the muscular prostration, become greater day by day. The vision grows dimmer; the local pains become more painful and more confirmed; and the sleeplessness at night becomes more and more distressing.

The symptoms which now assume a prominence, and which become connected, or engrafted as it were on the preceding phenomena, are — an intense thirst; a dry, parched, scaly skin; a voracious appetite; an excessive flow of urine of high specific gravity, which is highly charged with sugar; with increasing emaciation, which ultimately becomes extreme. Such is a brief outline of the leading symptoms of Diabetes Mellitus; but to complete the picture, it were well that we should dwell upon each a little more fully.

URINE. — Amongst the early and chief symptoms of Diabetes Mellitus which first claim our attention is an inordinate flow of urine. Indeed, it is by this symptom alone that the patient's attention is often first aroused to the fact that there is something wrong. He not only finds that he is called upon to micturate during the day oftener than he used to, but that he is obliged to leave his bed during the night for a like purpose: the quantity passed, also, he finds is wonderfully increased.

The actual quantity passed varies considerably in different cases, and according to the nature and stage of the complaint, and the mode of treatment adopted for its cure. The quantity of urine sometimes passed is positively enormous. P. Frank details a case in which 52 lbs. were passed in twenty-four hours. Pavy gives us the case of an out-door patient at Guy's Hospital, who ascertained, by measurement, that he was passing 20 quarts of urine a day. I have met with several cases of Diabetes within the last few years; one a very near relative, whose urine averaged about 20 pints a day; the specific gravity amounted to 1.050, which was reduced to its normal standard in eight weeks, by means of *Nux Vom, Podophyllum, Leptandra*, Turkish Baths, and a well-regulated diet. The second a lady, aged 37, who averaged 17 pints a day; the specific gravity did not exceed 1.035. The third case was that of a clergyman, aged 46, who voided about 19 pints a day; the specific gravity varied from 1.034 to 1.042. He was cured in three months. [1] Clinical history gives us many instances where it is by no means uncommon, that from 25 to 35 pints have been discharged in the same time, for weeks and even months together.

It a straightforward and uncomplicated case of Diabetes, the quantity of urine passed in a given time affords a fair index as to the amount of sugar passed at the same time. The specific gravity of Diabetic urine may reach as high as 1.050, or even a little higher, but the usual range is from 1.030 or 1.035 to 1.045; and when the disease has been checked by proper medical, hygienic, and dietetic treatment, the specific gravity may sink even below the normal standard.

Colour. — The colour of ordinary Diabetic urine is that of a pale-straw or greenish tint; this, however, varies with the quantity that is passed. Much also depends on diet and the time of day the urine is passed.

When the quantity passed is large, the urine is so pale as to approach that of spring water.

When the quantity of water is checked, the colour approaches that belonging to the healthy secretion. Urine passed at different periods during the twenty/four hours, presents a marked variation in colour. /

The urine passed on rising in the morning, is, as /a' rule, more highly coloured than what is passed in the course of the day, because, from the non-ingestion of food during the night, there is less sugar to I be eliminated, and the amount of fluid discharged is lessened accordingly. For the converse reason, the urine passed upon going to bed at night is usually found to be about the palest of any.

ODOUR. — Diabetic urine is to be distinguished from all other abnormal secretions of a like kind by its peculiar "Nose," and has been differently described by different authorities — (see page 37.)

CLEAENESS. — Freedom from turbidity is another and very characteristic feature of Diabetic urine. When the disease is severe, the urine is invariably bright and clear on cooling: but when the complaint is successfully brought under control, we find a copious deposit of lithates — an indication of returning health.

In concluding our remarks on the phenomena depicted in Diabetic urine, I may refer to the effect of the presence of sugar in causing white spots to be left on articles of clothing where drops of urine have fallen. Pavy and others have frequently noticed these spots on the boots and trousers of those afflicted with Diabetes Mellitus.

THIRST — or Poly-dipsia. — The existence of thirst, which is more or less persistent, and at times unquenchable, is another and very characteristic symptom of Diabetes. It is a very distressing thirst — a kind of thirst that cannot be quenched, however much fluid is taken. Patients have been astonished at the enormous quantity of water they have drank; and yet the thirst continues: they have often confessed to having emptied the contents of the water bottles, and even the ewer on the wash-stand, during the night, and have known not why? — the more they drank, the more they wanted to drink. This thirst is generally most intense towards evening, and through the night, and with the parched mouth and sleeplessness, renders the condition of the sufferer one of extreme wretchedness and distress. This fiery and unquenchable thirst from which the Diabetic complains of, is, however, readily accounted for upon simple physiological grounds; viz. — The sugar, in escaping from the system, carries with it water from the blood, and thus leaves the vital fluid in a more or less concentrated condition. Now, the solid and liquid matter of the blood ought to bear a certain normal relationship to each other; and to uphold this relationship, we have the action of the eliminative organs on the one hand, and a certain sensation on the other, which not only makes us conscious when fluid is required, but it excites us with a strong desire to take it. It matters little in what way the solid matter of the blood becomes out of proportion to the normal proportion of the liquid. Whether it be by the rapid escape of fluid through the skin by free perspiration following active exercise; — whether by the action of the vapour or Turkish Bath; — whether as in the case of pudlers when exposed to the heat of a fiery furnace; — whether by the ingestion of a quantity of saline matter, as from eating salt provisions; — or whether from deprivation of a proper supply of drink; — or whether it takes place from copious serous evacuations, as in Asiatic cholera or the disease we are now discussing; — in each case the result is the same — viz., a sensation is excited that we denominate THIEST, which has the effect of inducing us to take what is wanted to restore the balance that has been disarranged. Thus thirst is designed by a wise Providence for providing that the blood is supplied with a due and normal proportion of liquid; and such, indeed, is the strength of that wonderful sensation when fluid is urgently needed, that an irresistible desire to drink is excited — the voice of Nature appealing lustily for succour. Drink here is, in fact, replacing that fluid which is being so extensively discharged by the kidneys during the progress of the disease.

It is this persistent THIRST, coupled by a persistently copious discharge of URINE, which usually first excites, in the minds of the patients and their friends, suspicion that there is something radically wrong: and these two symptoms will often suffice to lead the practitioner to a safe and correct diagnosis.

MOUTH. — A dry, parched, clammy condition of the mouth, is another distressing phenomenon of Diabetes, and is invariably associated with thirst, which is not in the least degree assuaged by large and repeated draughts of cold water, or any other beverage: the lips are parched, and the angles of the mouth are bedewed with thick mucus: the tongue is also dry, unwieldly, and clings to the roof of the mouth. To those accustomed to be thrown much in contact with Diabetic patients, says Pavy, the state of the mouth alone will sometimes suffice to lead to the suspicion of the existence of the disease. The patient, as he is speaking, is constantly rolling the tongue in a peculiar manner about in the mouth, and passing it over the lips, apparently with the view of lubricating with what scanty moisture he has: and from sticking as it does to the roof of the mouth, on account of the great dryness that exists, a peculiar sound is produced, which is very significant and suggestive to those who have once given more than ordinary attention to it.

TONG-UE. — The appearance of this organ varies considerably in different cases: sometimes it is morbidly clean; sometimes it is morbidly red, and presents a strong resemblance to raw meat; sometimes it is covered with a white creamy fur; and at other times the fur is dry and brown, particularly in the advanced stage of the complaint.

BREATH and TASTE. — A peculiar aromatic odour emanates from the skin and lungs of Diabetic patients, which was first noticed by Latham. It, however, disappears as the disease is subdued by treatment, but again re-appears on the administration of anything which sends up the saccharine matter in the urine.

TEETH and GUMS.— A spongy, bleeding condition of the gums, and a loosened condition of the teeth, which sometimes fall out, is not an uncommon symptom of Diabetes. "There is," says Pavy, "some direct connection between this phenomenon and the disease. It seems as if the morbid condition of the system prevailing interfered with the nutritive action going on in the fang and its socket, and to lead to that result."

SKIN. — A dry and unperspiring condition of the skin is a marked feature of Diabetes, particularly in its advanced stage, and like the thirst and dried mouth, is produced by the continual abstraction from the system of the large quantity of water which is continually passing off by the kidneys. The insensible perspiration is enormously diminished; so much so, that according to the experiments of Von Dursch, only 200 grammes of water passed off by the skin and lungs in the twenty-four hours, instead of the normal quantity — namely, from 1 to 2,000 grammes, or ten ounces, instead of fifty to 100 ounces: and it is more than probable that the whole of the small quantity mentioned by Von Dursch escaped by the lungs; such is the hermetically sealed condition and inactivity of the skin under such circumstances.

DIGESTION. — The process of digestion varies considerably in Diabetics; in some cases, during the early stages, there is but little to complain of; in others a train of dyspeptic symptoms is set up, more or less severe: loss of appetite, a loathing for food, nausea, flatulence, eructations, and sickness sometimes prevail; which may constitute a prominent symptom. As the disease advances the appetite becomes abnormally increased, and an enormous quantity of food is consumed in the twenty-four hours. This inordinate appetite, which has been termed by Dr. Jaccoud, of Paris, Polyphagia ($\phi\acute{\alpha}\gamma\omega$, to eat), indicates the approach of the most serious phase of the complaint, when a considerable portion of the albuminoid principles of the food is converted into sugar, and eliminated by the urine. It consequently follows, that the intensity of the Polyphagia is one of the most prominent indexes we have of the extent of the mal-assimilation and saccharine metamorphosis of the nitrogenous alimentary substances destined for the healthy nutrition of the tissues of the body.

This misappropriation of the food of the tissues creates a corresponding want, which .in turn excites an inordinate appetite; hence the prominence of Polyphagia as a symptom of Diabetes. It may further be observed that this enormous appetite increases in intensity in proportion to the increased severity and advanced progress of the complaint; so that even enormous quantities of food — like the enormous quantity of fluids — are consumed by the patient without the thirst or the cravings and constant pangs of hunger ever being satisfied. Under these peculiar circumstances, it is a wise provision on the part of nature to retain the functions of digestion in a VIGOROUS and unimpaired condition, in order that inordinate quantity of food might be digested, which in the healthy subject might cause serious gastric derangement.

EMACIATION. — A gradual and uniform waste of tissues is another prominent and important symptom of Diabetes: the patient's fat and flesh vanishes, and the loss of weight in a very short time may be extreme. This symptom did not escape the observation of the ancient physicians, as Aretseus, in his admirable description of the disease, designates it as a "Wonderful affection, being a melting down of the flesh and limbs into urine." This forms the fifth important symptom, as described by Dr. Jaccoud, and designated by him Auto-phagia. The precise period at which the emaciation begins, varies in different cases, being regulated more or less by the intensity of the disease, and other conditions. In the first stage of the disease the emaciation is marked by the gradual disappearance of the adipose tissue; this after a time is followed by a wasting of the flesh, till the patient is reduced to a mere skeleton.

DEBILITY.— Following that condition of the body termed Auto-phagia is debility, which is complained of to a far greater extent than what can be accounted for by the emaciation present. It is one of the early symptoms of the disease, which becomes more confirmed day by day as the disease advances,

VIRILITY. — During the course of the disease the power and function of re-production are more or less suspended in both sexes, but which returns as vigorously as ever on the removal of the Diabetes.

CRAMPS. — A spasmodic contraction of the muscles of the legs forms a no uncommon symptom of Diabetes; it generally occurs at night, while in bed, and gives rise to considerable pain and inconvenience: this, however, like other symptoms disappears on the removal of the sugar from the system.

DROPSY. — Puffiness of the lower limbs, particularly around the ankles, may be looked upon as an occasional symptom of Diabetes. It is, however, of little importance, unless complicated with fatty degeneration of the kidneys. We well know that Bright's Disease is sometimes associated with Diabetes, and will, when existing alone, give rise to dropsical effusion in the legs: this is easily ascertained by testing for "albumen," which is invariably found connected with Bright's Disease, in the urine: and if present gives rise to the most serious consequences.

CONSTIPATION.— From the extensive and continued loss of fluid through the kidneys, the system is deprived of its diluting and lubricating properties; hence an unnaturally dry and hard consistency of the contents of the large intestines, which render their expulsion exceedingly difficult and painful. To this rule, however, there are exceptions, as the very opposite condition sometimes happens; as it may occur that, as constipation is overcome, a diarrhoea sets in, and so on in alternation, to the great annoyance and inconvenience of the patient.

Such are the leading phenomena connected with a well-marked case of Diabetes; but to complete the picture there are certain other manifestations it would be well briefly to dwell upon, and which will take their place under the head of

COMPLICATIONS. — Amongst the most common of these, is a chronic form of pulmonary disease, usually spoken of as Phthisis; but although it runs the same course, and presents the same symptoms as " Tubercular Phthisis," yet it seems in reality to constitute a result of "simple chronic inflammatory action," attended with a break-down of the lung tissue and the formation of cavities, and to all appearances unconnected altogether with any strumous diathesis or tubercular deposit. But the frequency of this condition is such, that Copland scarcely met with a case of Diabetes which was entirely uncomplicated with pulmonic symptoms. Similar remarks have been made by Bardsley and others; and on this account, it may be inferred that the appellation given to the disease by Nicolas and Gruendeville, of PHTHISURIE SUCREE is a very appropriate one. Pavy regards this form of lung disease as a chronic inflammatory action, dependent on the presence of such an amount of sugar in the blood as to alter its natural quality, and to render it unfit for the healthy discharge of its functions.

CARBUNCLES, BOILS and GANGRENE.— These very painful and alarming complications are frequently met with in cases of Diabetes, and sometimes constitute the immediate cause of a fatal issue. The two former generally appear during the course of the second stage of the disease; are slow and painful in their development, and when suppuration takes place, are slow to heal. The latter generally appears at the close of the scene. This is not at all incomprehensible, seeing the great derangement to the process of interstitial nutrition, to which a supersaturated saccharine condition of the blood gives rise.

COMA. — Amongst the harbingers of death which usher in the closing scene of Diabetes, is that profound drowsiness or lethargic sleep termed " Coma." It is generally preceded by great weakness and prostration, a quick and feeble pulse, irritability of the stomach, which may even amount to vomiting. The intellect becomes blunted, and soon Coma gradually sets in, and becomes more and more profound, until the pulse is no longer felt. This condition appears as though it resulted from the effects of blood-poisoning; and looking upon it in this light, the term GLYCOHAEMIA might not inaptly be applied upon like grounds that Uraemia is employed to comprehend the analogous train of phenomena which frequently occur in connection with the closing scene of Bright's Disease.

CATARACT. — Before quitting this part of our subject, there is one more symptom to be referred to, which is worthy of note; that is, the frequent association of Cataract with Diabetes. This interesting fact has of late attracted considerable attention from physiologists, on account of its having been discovered — by experiments on the lower animals — that Cataract may be produced by the introduction of sugar into the system. Diabetic Cataract has been noticed by Prout, Pavy, and France, of Guy's Hospital and by myself. It is, however, to Dr. S. W. Mitchell, an American physician, that we are indebted for first pointing out that sugar is capable of producing Cataract.

ECZEMA. — Another symptom, but little known or seldom recognised as one of the phenomena of Diabetes Mellitus, is an eczematous condition of the lower part of the abdomen, the vulva, and inner surface of the thighs in women; the orifice of the urethra and corona glandis in men. This symptom has, however, been recognised, more or less frequently, by Dickinson, Pavy, Wiltshire, Braxton Hicks, Trousseau, and myself. Dickinson, in his able treatise on Diabetes, notices the eczematous condition of the vulva as peculiar to the disease, and may be looked upon as one of the first signs by which the disease may be diagnosed.

J. Braxton Hicks affirms, that as many as eight or nine out of every ten women who consult him at Guy's Hospital on account of eczema of the genitals, are subjects of Diabetes Mellitus, as he has invariably found the urine heavily charged with saccharine matter. " Before," says Hicks, " I had been in the habit of examining the urine of every case of this kind, I had a patient of about fifty years of age, some years of whose life were scarcely tolerable on account of this form of eczema, and who had been treated by all the remedies for that complaint. After two or three years, she said to me, 'I do not know if it is of any importance to tell you, but I was, many years ago, pronounced to have a mild condition of Diabetes.' I then examined her urine frequently, and found always full evidence of sugar."

The eminently practical Trousseau, of Paris, says — "With this perversion of the functions of the skin, coincides another accident, which has been observed rarely in men, but much more commonly in women. It is an eczematous eruption attacking the genitals, and which is attended by a very distressing itching. When, in women of some age, you find this eczema, not dependent on the leucorrhoea, nor on menstruation, then our ideas should flow towards glycosuria." A somewhat extensive experience in Diabetes, enables me to record fifteen cases in women in whom this distressing symptom was very prominently marked. They expressed to me, without an exception, the restless nights and torments they had endured for months and months, which rendered life a heavy burden, and almost unbearable. The majority had been treated allopathically for simple eczema; five had consulted eminent dermatologists for a like purpose, neither of whom suspected the "fons et origo" of the eczematous eruption. They were all treated by me for Diabetes; thirteen were rapidly cured; two were obstinate, and required some months', close and careful watching.

[1] These patients came to consult me from North Wales.

Chapter Six - Physiology of Diabetes Mellitus

IF we desire," says Harley, " to be philosophical as well as practical, it is necessary that we should thoroughly understand both the origin and destruction of the sugar met with in the animal economy." For this purpose we will proceed briefly to consider the physiological phenomena of Diabetes Mellitus.

We may *in limine* observe, that sugar forms a normal constituent of the human body, and the escape of which from the system with the urine forms one of the most characteristic symptoms of Diabetes; it moreover constitutes a material which enters largely into the composition of our food, and plays an important part in the animal economy. That sugar is a natural constituent of the human frame is fully established by the experiments of Bruke, Bence Jones, Harley, Pavy, and others. This is easily shown by the following simple chemical process. Withdraw an ounce of blood from the arm of a healthy man in full digestion; allow it to fall drop by drop into a couple of ounces of boiling water, faintly acidulated with *acetic acid*. By this process all the albuminous matters are so firmly coagulated, that on filtration a perfectly colourless fluid is obtained, and on now applying to it the copper-potash, or fermentation tests, the existence of sugar becomes clearly perceptible.

SECONDLY. — Sugar as an *alimentary* principle is derived from the vegetable kingdom — cane sugar — and forms an abundant commercial product. Its properties are exceedingly soluble and -diffusible; requires no preparatory digestive process for its absorption; and passes readily from the alimentary canal into the blood-vessels ramifying upon its villous surface; according to the law of Osmosis. From these it is conducted, — not at once into the general circulation, as is the case with the matters absorbed by the lacteals,— but through the PORTAL SYSTEM of veins, direct into the liver. This is a physiological fact of great importance, for it has been shown by a series of experimental inquiries, that the liver arrests the sugar, and transforms it into a new body, which has received the name of amyloid substance.

THIRDLY. — There is another substance in our food which bears a strong analogy to sugar, and which is found far more extensively diffused throughout the vegetable world than the cane sugar; this product is STARCH, which is changed into saccharine matter by means of the SALIVA, the digestive and pancreatic juices. All foods coming from the vegetable kingdom — and of these the cereals are the most important — viz., wheat, barley, oats, rye, maize, Indian corn, rice, millet, and Guinea corn; secondly, the various pulses — peas, beans, lentils, and the dholls and grains of India; and thirdly, arrow-root, tapioca, cassava, sago, potatoes, turnips, carrots, parsnips, &c., contain a large quantity of starch, which starch, during its passage along the alimentary canal, is all, or nearly so, converted into sugar through the agency of the digestive juices, more particularly the PTYALINE of the saliva, and the pancreatin of the pancreatic fluid, as likewise by the animal diastase of intestinal mucus. The solution is effected by the conversion of the *starchy* and *cellulose* properties into a low form of sugar, called *glucose,* which is either freely absorbed into the circulation, or is changed in the stomach into lactic acid, where it serves an important function in the digestion of nitrogenous matter. If, however, by mal-assimilation, through the agency perhaps of putrefactive processes, it becomes changed into butyric acid, it hinders digestion, and causes much discomfort. It is on this account that saccharine foods are apt to disagree with the stomach; and it is very probable that this abnormal transformation is due to the presence of those infusorial creatures which swarm in putrefying animal matters.

The transformation of starchy (amylaceous) matters into glucose (sugar) during the period they tarry in the alimentary canal, is not — says Harley — the result of accident, but the sequence of a natural law, which is equally in force in or out of the body, so long as the physical conditions necessary for its action are in operation. This may be illustrated by the following chemical process: — Place an ounce of boiled arrowroot in a test-tube; add to this a little saliva and a few drops of pancreatic juice; in a few minutes the whole of the starch contained in the arrowroot will be turned into sugar: and the only agency used for this purpose is a temperature equal to that of the human body. As regards carnivorous animals, a similar change occurs; and the sugar thus formed is absorbed by the mesenteric veins and lacteals, and forms part of that met with in the circulation.

In illustration of this fact. Professor Sharpey, and Harley, of University College Hospital, drew from the femoral artery of a dog which had been previously fed for four days on boiled flesh, and perfectly devoid of sugar, two ounces of blood, which was allowed to flow directly into boiling water slightly acidulated with acetic acid; and when the clear filtrate from this blood was tested it yielded clear traces of sugar, which sugar must have been formed in the animal's body, seeing that not a particle of sugar was introduced with the food. This experiment is conclusive that the animal system contains a sugar-manufacturing organ; and Nature has in her munificence supplied us with proofs: and this doubtless exists in all animals, whether they be purely carnivorous, herbivorous, or those that partake of a mixed diet. The Polar bear not only lives on animal diet, but on the flesh of animals, such as the walrus and seal, whose chief food is fish, which fish, in their turn, are *not supposed to live on vegetables;* and yet this bear feeds her young with her own milk, which undoubtedly holds in solution saccharine matter. The more advanced physiologists of the present day maintain that the carnivorous animal has the power of forming sugar out of albuminous substances; and in the case of the herbivorous animal, the sugar met with in its milk is not directly obtained from the digestive canal. This is fairly proved by the following illustrations.

Milk sugar possesses certain properties which distinguish it from all vegetable sugars.

Milk sugar, although abundantly present in milk, has not yet been detected in the general circulation. The natural conclusion therefore is, that the mammary gland acts as a manufacturing organ: consequently there must be, in every body, one organ capable of forming saccharine matter.

We now approach that stage of our investigation when it becomes necessary to ask the question — In what organ of the body is the sugar formed which is met with in the general circulation of the carnivora? The answer is, the liver. And why? The blood of carnivora proceeding to the liver is devoid of sugar; but that coming from the liver is highly charged with sugar. This has been proved by a series of experiments made by Bernard, Harley, and Schmidt, the results of which are as follows: —

	Per-centage of sugar in	
	Portal vein.	Hepatic vein.
First dog fed on animal diet	0.00	0.93
Second ,, ,, ,,	0.00	0.99
Third ,, fasting during two days	0.00	0.51

These results, which have been fully confirmed by the extensive experiments performed by Pavy, go far to furnish us with the key to that well-known fact, that some Diabetic patients, even when totally restricted to animal diet, still pass a large quantity of sugar.

Having now ascertained, by clear and unmistakable evidence, that the healthy blood always contains sugar, and that when the saccharine matter is not obtained from without, the body under these circumstances sets up its own "manufactory" and generates it for itself; the next step for our consideration is, to ascertain whether sugar is essentially required to support life; and if so, to what use or uses is it put to, to sustain the animal organism.; and whether the quantity of sugar in the blood is always the same in quantity, or liable to variation, and to what extent. Upon this point, which has been ascertained by a series of experiments made by several of the leading experimental physiologists of the present day, the amount of saccharine matter found in the arterial blood of healthy animals is subject to great variation; viz., from an almost inappreciable quantity after long fasting, up to 0.24 per cent, during the time of full digestion. Bernard found as much as 2 per cent, in the hepatic vein. From this it may be inferred that the quantity of sugar present in the general circulation follows a general law — it increases in quantity as digestion advances, and gradually diminishes as the time approaches for the next meal, — the maximum being reached four hours after food, the minimum on fasting. This variation in the amount of sugar found in the circulation according to the condition and stage of the digestion, affords to the physician a key, whereby he is able to account for the fluctuation which takes place in the amount of sugar found in the urine of Diabetic patients in the course of twenty-four hours; and it also explains why, in some slight cases of Diabetes, saccharine matter is only found in the urine a few hours after a meal. It must, however, be borne in mind that the amount of sugar in the blood not only fluctuates according to the stage of the digestion, but that it varies considerably in proportion to the quality and the quantity of food taken. To illustrate this, Professor Sharpey, of University College Hospital, fed three dogs on horse-flesh; four hours afterwards he drew some blood from each of their carotid arteries, which only yielded on an average 0.08 per cent, of sugar. Whereas when the same dogs were fed on a mixed diet consisting of *potatoes, meat,* and *bread,* the saccharine matter in the same fluid rose to 0.22 per cent. — a conclusive proof that a purely animal diet diminishes, whilst a vegetable or mixed diet increases, the amount of sugar eliminated by the kidneys. Another physiological fact worth recording at this stage of our investigation is, that although the quantity of sugar present in the circulation is constantly fluctuating, the amount found in the liver remains comparatively unaltered. Harley accounts for this as follows: — " The reason why the amount of saccharine matter remains comparatively stationary in the liver while it is constantly fluctuating in the circulation, arises from the circumstance of the sugar not being stored up in the hepatic cells, but poured into the vessels as quickly as it is formed; therefore the quantity which the liver at any time contains cannot be accepted as a criterion of the amount which the organ produces."

Having so far traced the *rationale* of sugary urine, we have now to ascertain whether animal food is directly transformed into sugar; or whether there is a kind of TRANSITION STAGE between the protein substance (in the form of a rump-steak) on the one hand, and saccharine matter on the other hand. We have already made ourselves acquainted with the fact, that in the case of starchy or amylaceous substances, there exists no connecting link or transitional stage whatever; but that during their progress along the intestinal canal, they come into contact with certain digestive and solvent juices, which at once convert them into sugar, in which condition it is carried direct into the liver.

FIRSTLY — These solvent juices consist, as I have already pointed out, of *ptyalin,* which is a nitrogenous substance, of the nature of *diastase* — the ferment which in the vegetable converts starch into sugar; and hence it has been called animal diastase by Mialhe, who attaches great importance to it as the principal agent concerned in the digestion of starchy foods; one part of ptyalin, according to him, being capable of converting 8,000 parts of insoluble starch into soluble glucose. Saliva, of which ptyalin is its active principle, has no chemical action on FAT, fibrin, or ALBUMINOUS substances — its real functions being, to lubricate the food for deglutition, to carry oxygen into the stomach, and more particularly, to furnish a solvent for starch and tender cellulose. Those animals, therefore, that feed chiefly on woody matters, as the beaver, and most of the rodent animals, have large salivary glands: besides this, provision is likewise made for a prolonged contact of the ptyalin with the vegetable tissue, in order to ensure its complete transformation.

THE SECOND of these solvent juices is pancreatin, the active principle of the pancreatic fluid — a colourless liquid of specific gravity 1.008 or 1.009, derived from the pancreas, or sweetbread. Pancreatin has not only the remarkable property of converting starchy substances into sugar, but it has also the same remarkable property of breaking down the larger granules, crystals, and globules of oil and fat into myriads of smaller globules of from the 1-3,000 to the 1-15,000 of an inch in diameter. In this way the fat is emulsified, and converted into a milky fluid, which mixes freely with water, and passes through the tissues of the intestines into the lacteals. Pancreatin is therefore a powerful agent of digestion, in so far as fat, starch, and young cellulose are concerned: but it has little or no action on albuminous substances.

THE THIRD of these solvent juices is the Bile; and although the true functions of this secretion still remain more or less in obscurity, yet it is more than probable that it aids in neutralising the acid peptones from the stomach; in emulsifying the fat; in helping the digestion of starchy food; and more particularly in the conversion of amylaceous substances into saccharine matter. With proteinaceous substances, however, the case assumes a very different aspect; for ere they can be changed into saccharine matter, they must first undergo a "chemical change" which converts the substance into something like starch. The more, indeed, we study, and penetrate deeper and deeper into the hitherto dark and mysterious laws of nature, the more — when that curtain is removed — are we forced to admire the beneficence, uniformity, and wondrous applicability of those laws. In the vegetable as well as in the animal kingdoms, we not only encounter similar substances, but we likewise find that they are endowed with similar properties, and perform similar functions. The cane sugar has its simile in the sugar of the milk; the grape sugar has its simile in the sugar of the liver; and even so the vegetable starch, as will be seen, has its simile in the animal world.

Simile gaudet simili.

Like will to like.
The grasshopper, we find, befriends the grasshopper.
The careful ant befriends the ant.
The very hawkes befriend the hawkes: but me the Muses.

- *Theocritus Idils, x. b. 31. &c.*
282 B.C.

39

It was in 1848 that Claude Bernard first discovered that the liver was a sugar-producing organ, and that without any vegetable principle being concerned. In 1857 he was enabled to announce, that the isolation of the sugar-forming material had been effected, and that such material bore a strong resemblance to starch; in consequence of which he gave to this newly discovered product the name of "Griucogene," which is another name for " starch sugar " — from the Greek γλυκὺς, sweet. — Others designate it as Amyloid matter, or Hepatine (Pavy); and Zoamyline by Rouget: but for the sake of perspicuity, we will, on further investigating this subject, adhere to Bernard's nomenclature of Glucogene.

ANATOMICALLY, Olucogene has its seat in the hepatic cells, and according to Hensen is of a yellow colour, easily transformable into sugar by means of saliva, pancreatic juice, and even portal blood. CHEMICALLY, Griucogene presents alliances to both starch and dextrine, but resembles the latter more strongly than the former. Like these substances it constitutes a neutral, colourless, or slightly yellow, tasteless, inodorous, and uncrystallisable body. It is soluble in water, and presents this peculiarity — In a small quantity of water it is transparent; in a large quantity it becomes milky; it is insoluble in alcohol and acetic acid. When boiled with diluted mineral acids, or treated with either saliva, pancreatic juice, blood, or liver tissue, it is transformed like other starchy substances into sugar of the second class. With the tincture of Iodine it yields a deep winered colour: and as long as it exists as pure Glucogene, it yields no reaction with the copper, fermentation, or any other sugar test.

To extract the Glucogene substance from the liver the following simple process will suffice. Let a piece of the organ taken from a recently killed healthy animal be plunged for a few minutes into boiling water, so as to destroy the ferment that is present and prevent any further loss of the substance by transformation into sugar. It is then to be well pounded in a mortar, treated with a moderate quantity of water, and thoroughly boiled. The decoction thus procured, after having been strained or filtered, is poured into about five or six times its bulk of spirit, by means of which the Grlucogene substance is thrown down as a dense white precipitate. This may now be collected on a filter, washed with spirit, and dried.

Glucogene is a substance which, according to E. Pelouse, belongs to the Carbo-Hydrate group; is devoid of nitrogen; and gives as its formula $C_{12} H_{12} O_{12}$ which is derived from the following analysis: —

Carbon ...   39.8
Hydrogen ...   6.1
Oxygen ...   54.1
                100.0

Dr. Odling, of Guy's Hospital, gives the four following specimens, as his analysis of Glucogenic substances procured from the livers of rabbits.

Specimen No. 1. — Prepared by precipitation, and washing with alcohol only, yielded —

Carbon ...   42.68
Hydrogen ...   6.47
Oxygen   ... 50.32
Nitrogen ...   0.53
                    100.00

Specimen No. 2. — Precipitated and washed with spirit, after having been boiled with dilute hydrochloric acid, yielded —

Carbon ...   43.24
Hydrogen ...   6.38
Oxygen ...   49.99
Nitrogen ...   0.39
                    100.00

Specimen No. 3. — Prepared in the same way as No. 2, excepting that it was boiled with glacial acetic acid, instead of hydrochloric acid. This yielded —

Carbon ...   42.80
Hydrogen ...   6.15
Oxygen ...   50.58
Nitrogen...   0.47
                    100.00

Specimen No. 4. — Treated by boiling with a strong solution of potash for half an hour, and then precipitated and washed with alcohol, which yielded —

Carbon ...   42.97
Hydrogen ...   6.63
Oxygen ...   50.29
Nitrogen ...   0.11
                    100.00

Professor Apjohn, of Dublin, confirms the above analysis by the following, as also prepared from the livers of rabbits — viz.:

Carbon ...   43.78
Hydrogen ...   6.32
Oxygen ...   49.28
Nitrogen ...   0.62
                    100.00

Glucogene has been detected in the livers of all animals in which it has hitherto been sought after, no matter whether they were animal or vegetable feeders, cold or warm blooded. The oyster and mussel is charged with a large quantity of it: and not only does the liver of the mussel contain this Glucogene, but the entire mantle is richly charged with it when the animal is in a good and healthy condition: but when poor, as after spawning, the mantle is thin, transparent, watery, and contains but little Glucogene. When under an opposite condition, the mantle of the animal is thick, and opaquely white, or yellowish, and in such a condition is highly charged with glucogenic matter, which seems to form a kind of store, to be drawn upon during the season of spawning. No sugar has been detected in the mantle at the time of death: the addition of saliva, however, is immediately followed by the formation of saccharine matter.

We now approach that part of our investigation when it becomes necessary to ask the question, What are the uses of Glucogene in the animal economy — simply in its natural form?

"It is well known to all," says Harley, "that starch, simply as starch, cannot nourish the body: it is therefore more than probable that Griucogene must, like ordinary starchy matter, be transformed into saccharine matter before it can play its part in the intricate processes of life. From all that has been known, the greater part of the Glucogene formed in the liver is changed into sugar ere it leaves that organ; and whatever the transforming agency may be, it is something foreign and independent of the so-called vital influences. The transformation of Glucogene into sugar appears to follow the same unalterable law as that which effects the transformation of common starch; and not only does it continue in force after the death of the animal, but even after the removal of the liver from the body: all that is required, apparently, being the sustaining the organ at a certain temperature." This has been amply proved by the experiments of C. Bernard, and many others who have followed him in similar investigations.

The next question to be answered is, What becomes of all the sugar when formed, and whence its destination? Claude Bernard thought that it was burned off in the lungs, its chief office being to sustain animal heat. Dr. McDonnell propounded an idea that the Glucogene becomes blended with nitrogen in the liver, and leaves the organ through the hepatic veins as a "proteic compound;" partly, he thinks, in the form of globuline, caseine, or albuminoss. He further thinks that the liver does for the adult what divers tissues do during the development of the foetus. " May not this great organ," says he, "with the help of the Glucogene substance secreted in its cells, form a nitrogenous compound, just as the muscles of the foetus convert the Glucogene contained in them into the highly nitrogenous materials of muscular tissue? And may not the glucogenic substance of the liver be the basis of an azotized protoplasma, forming a constituent of the blood of the adult animal, as the Glucogene substance of muscle is the basis of the material from which the evolution of muscular tissues is accomplished? "

Pavy is of opinion that the glucogenic substance goes to the manufacture of fat; for it has been ascertained beyond dispute, that starch and sugar, introduced with the food, lead, in the animal system, to the production of fat: and it has been further shown, that, from the ingestion of these principles, a striking increase is developed in the amount of glucogenic substances contained in the liver. The production of Glucogene, therefore, may be taken as representing the first step of assimilation of the starchy and saccharine elements of our food; and, as these elements are known to proceed on into adipose tissue, we have strong grounds for surmising that the Glucogene simply occupies an intermediate post between the two. This process of assimilation may go on to the production of fat in the liver; or, it may be, that it stops short, at the incipient stage, of the formation of another principle, which escapes from the liver, and is elsewhere transformed into fat, by means perhaps of the biliary secretion. Chauveau, Harley, and others agree in substance with Pavy, and that the saccharine matter disappears in the capillaries of the general circulation; — further confirmed by experiments that less sugar is found in the veins returning from the extremities of limbs than exists in the arteries going to it: and from its thus disappearing in the capillaries, we are naturally led to infer that this substance plays an important part in the nutritive process of the animal economy. Negroes, it is said, become fat and indolent during the sugar-harvest, from sucking the young, fresh, and juicy cane, which they undoubtedly do in large quantities, as witnessed by myself on a sugar estate on the banks of the Demerara. Babies fatten on sugar quicker than anything else: cats and dogs soon become fat and sleek on the same substance. Oxen and sheep prepared for the Christmas show, have no other food than oil-cake, mangel-wurzel, beet-root, turnips, and a little hay: and pigs, barley-meal and a little milk, which make the finest and most delicious bacon. A very near relative has, for years past, accustomed himself to a bason of GRUEL as a nightcap. He gradually grew fatter, and is now looked upon as a second Tichborne, and may ultimately vie with a Daniel Lambert.

We have long been taught that bees have the power of transforming sugar into wax. We are now being made acquainted with the startling fact, that man and other animals have a sugar-manufacturing organ, which goes to furnish the system with adipose matter.

Chapter Seven - Pathology of Diabetes

HAVING now touched upon, and disposed of, some of the leading and most important points connected with the physiology of Diabetes, our next step will be to consider another and still more important section of our discourse — namely, its "pathological phases." We may *in limine* observe, that

Diabetes Mellitus is one of the most intricate diseases which comes across the path of the anxious physician, as it but seldom leaves in its wake any prominent landmarks, or anatomical lesions, whereby a clue can be obtained of the "fons et origo" of the malady; and which would act as a polar star for his future guidance and treatment. Physicians of the past century have attributed Diabetes to organic changes in the kidneys, the ureters, and bladder; the splanchnic nerves; the liver, stomach, and intestines; the spleen and pancreas; and the lungs and heart. But these, as many recent observers contend, are rather its effects than its causes. It is not, therefore, within the precincts of the dead-house, but at the bed-side of the patient, in the clinical ward, the physiological and chemical laboratory, that the nature, cause, and treatment of this mysterious affection is most successfully studied and combated. Indeed, we shall soon find, that the intense thirst; the inordinate appetite; the dry and parched skin; the gradual emaciation of the body; and the inordinate flow of urine " of high specific gravity," and holding in solution more or less saccharine matter — like the orange-coloured skin in Jaundice — are merely signals, landmarks, or outward manifestations of several widely-differing abnormal conditions of the system; the correct appreciation and knowledge of which will entirely depend on our acquaintance with its physiology.

Claude Bernard, as the result of his investigations and interesting experiments, came to the conclusion that the excessive formation of sugar, "constituting Diabetes Mellitus," arose from a disordered innervation of the liver, produced from some cause situated in some part of the brain. This conclusion he arrived at by discovering that a saccharine condition of the urine can be induced by puncturing the floor of the fourth ventricle of the brain, near the origin of the pneumogastric nerves. ANATOMICALLY, this ventricle is triangular in shape; the front, or base, is formed by the medulla oblongata and "pons varolii;" the upper wall by the valve of Vieussens; the posterior wall by the cerebellum, and the continuation of the arachnoid membrane on the back of the spinal cord. The liver, therefore, may be considered as the organ which we must look to in Diabetes for the source of the sugar that appears in the blood, and thence is discharged with the urine: for it has been shown, in our physiological investigations, that it is the duty of the liver to *detain*, and convert into another principle, the sugar derived from the food, and absorbed from the alimentary canal. Sugar forms one of the natural elements of our food. It is absorbed from the digestive canal by the portal vessels, and carried to the liver. Should it pass direct through the liver, and enter the general circulation, it is then discharged in its normal condition from the system with the urine. Under natural circumstances, however, such a result does not take place: for the sugar is stopped by the liver, and retained till its properties are transformed or assimilated in such a manner as to render it better adapted to the purposes of life.

According to the views of C. Bernard, the sugar taken as food, or formed from starch during the process of digestion, becomes, after absorption into the vena cavae, first converted into Glucogene by the action of the secreting function of the liver cells, and afterwards changed, by a ferment-diastase, into sugar, or glucose, which, entering the general circulation, is conveyed to the lungs, and there destroyed by the oxygen inhaled from without. This doctrine of the combustion which the sugar undergoes in the lungs, was first suggested by the late Baron Liebig; but has since been set aside as untenable by Pavy and others. Pavy, by a series of careful and important investigations, confirms the correctness of the views advanced by C. Bernard, but disputes his conclusions. He denies that the liver is a sugar-manufacturing organ, and arrives at the following conclusions: —

1. That during life, as a natural condition, no sugar is found in the liver, or secreted by that organ.

2. That normally, during life, scarcely any Glucogene is transformed into sugar and taken up by the blood in its passage through the liver, in consequence of its colloidal character rendering it incapable of dialising through animal membranes.

3. That the sugar found so bountifully after death in the liver, and in the blood of that portion of the circulation intervening between it and the lungs, is produced by *post-mortem* changes and the development of a ferment in the liver itself; and that the evidence on which it was believed that the liver exercises a sugar-forming function, was based on conditions occurring after death, and differing essentially from those existing during life. Many attempts have been made to discover the source of the ferment which C. Bernard supposed to be required to transform the Glucogene in the liver into sugar; but no satisfactory results have hitherto followed.

Pavy believes that there are two distinct types of Diabetes. Harley is of the same opinion; and that one arises from excessive formation of sugar; the other from defective assimilation — malnutrition.

In those resulting from excessive formation, Pavy thinks there must be something abnormal in addition to the want of assimilative power over sugar, inasmuch as the urine continues to be saccharine even when starch and sugar are carefully excluded from the food: and to account for this occurrence, he considers we must look to the glucogenic substance existing in an abnormal quantity in the liver, as reasonably constituting the source of the sugar in the urine; this substance being exceedingly prone to undergo a downward metamorphosis into saccharine matter. Normally, this transformation is prevented from taking place to more than what the natural laws of nature dictate; but, under a variety of unnatural or abnormal circumstances, it is more or less freely allowed to take place; and, as a consequence, sugar appears to a corresponding extent in the general circulation, and proportionately so in the urine: HENCE DIABETES.

These unnatural or abnormal conditions of the system, which lead to the transformation of Glucogene into sugar, may be conveniently considered under the three following heads: —

Firstly. Lesions of the nervous system.

Secondly. A congested condition of the bloodvessels of the liver.

Thirdly. A change in the quality of the blood.

A. It is now a well-recognised and established fact, that the various secreting organs of the animal body are urged to perform their different functions by means of a direct and a reflex action of the nervous system; and the liver is not exempt from this law. Clinical observations, pathological researches, and physiological experiments, daily prove that an abnormal state of the brain or the severance of a special nerve, is followed by a non-saccharine condition of the urine. — Claude Bernard punctured the medulla oblongata of a frog, which was followed by sugar in the urine.

Schiff performed a similar operation on six frogs, with like results.

Harley severed the pneumogastric nerve in the neck, when the glucogenic function of the liver was immediately arrested. He afterwards applied galvanism to the UPPER ends of the severed nerves, which was followed by a restoration of the saccharine matter. This was effected by reflex action: the nerve force first travelled along the upper severed ends of the pneumogastric nerves to the brain; from thence it reflected along the spinal cord, splanchnic nerves, and great solar plexus, and from thence to the liver. To produce this effect, it is not absolutely necessary to apply the galvanism to the cervical portion of the pneumogastric nerve; for according to the duality of nerve-force, as first pointed out to us by the brilliant experimental discoveries of Marshall Hall, irritation produced at any point of a reflex nerve-circuit, is invariably followed by the same phenomena. C. Bernard enumerates three effects as capable of being produced upon the urine by puncture of the medulla oblongata, according to the exact spot that happens to form the seat of lesion — namely, GLUCOGENE, Polyuria, and Albuminuria; and although these effects may be conjoined, still they may occur singly — clearly showing their independence of each other. He states, that when the puncture is made in the median line of the fourth ventricle, midway between the origin of the pneumogastric and auditory nerves, both glycosuria and polyuria are produced; that when the puncture, on the other hand, is made a little higher up, the urine is less abundant and less charged with sugar, but found often to contain albumen; and when it is made a little below the origin of the auditory nerves, there is an augmentation in the quantity of urine, without the passage either of sugar or albumen.

Looking, then, at the results of these experiments — which, if space permitted, might be greatly extended — we cannot but arrive at the conclusion, that from the medulla oblongata an influence arises which, in some manner or other, affects the normal or abnormal position of the glucogenic substance contained in the liver in a marked degree; and further, that the medulla oblongata enjoys a power, in reference to this matter, which is not possessed either by the cerebrum or medulla spinalis. Now, it was whilst engaged in prosecuting this inquiry, that Dr. Pavy came down upon the fact, that *a strongly saccharine condition of the urine* rapidly follows injury or division of certain portions of the sympathetic system of nerves.

Clinical records, which extend from a far-off epoch to the present time, give us examples that Diabetes Mellitus has been known to follow —

1. Injury of some kind or other to the head, with or without fracture of the skull.

2. It has been known to follow a clot of blood which was found encircling the medulla oblongata and pons varolii. This was in the case of a man who was received into University College Hospital in 1859, in a state of insensibility, from which he never recovered. Sugar was found abundantly in the urine.

3. It has been known to follow external injury to the head. This was in the case of a woman who had hemiplegia and rigidity of the right side, the result of a fall down stairs. The specific gravity of her urine was 1.021, and contained strong traces of sugar. She recovered. — A similar case occurred in the practice of Dr. Goolden: it was that of a railway stoker, who was struck on the back part of his head by the handle of a crane: Diabetes remained a prominent symptom during his illness. Dr. Harley mentions the case of a medical man in Kent, who had suffered from Diabetes for a considerable time before the nature of the complaint was suspected: his urine was loaded with sugar, and of a specific gravity 1.044. The only cause attributable to this case was, that four years previously he had been thrown from his horse, and in some way or other got his head bent forwards; and for some time afterwards he could not turn the head either way without considerable pain; besides, the sense of smelling and hearing was considerably blunted.

4. Pavy relates a case of intense Diabetes which immediately followed a violent blow upon the head. It was that of a soldier, who, whilst undergoing his military exercises at Sandhurst, received a blow upon the head from the ramrod of a piece of artillery, which rendered him insensible for some time. C. Bernard remarks, that falls upon the head have been known to be followed by Diabetes, and directs attention to the case of a quarry-man who became Diabetic in this way; and, as recovery took place, the saccharine matter disappeared from the urine at the same time.

The same authority relates another case. It was that of a little girl, of four years old only, who was run over in the street: she was taken up insensible, and remained so until her death. Her respiration was convulsive or sobbing, but not stertorous; blood ran from the nose and mouth. A *post-mortem* revealed fracture of base of the skull, with corresponding brain bruises; the fornix and floor of the fourth ventricle was also bruised, with effusion of bloody serum in the ventricles. On testing for sugar, as much as five and a-half grains in the fluid ounce, with slight traces of albumen, were found.

In the *"Archives Générales de Médecine,"* t. xx., 1862, Fischer has placed together a number of cases, gathered from various sources, in which Diabetes Mellitus has been known to follow traumatic lesions of the brain. In twenty-one cases thus collected: —

4, Consisted of Polyuria without sugar — Diabetes Insipidus.

3, Polyuria with slight traces of sugar.

6, Temporary Glycosuria.

8, Permanent, or confirmed Diabetes Mellitus.

Arranged according to seat of injury: —

6, Resulted from blows upon the forehead.

5, From blows on the top and sides of the head.

5, From blows on the back part of the head. In the remaining five the seat of injury was undetermined.

Diabetes has been known to follow Epilepsy, from disease of the pons varolii, and calamus scriptorius of the fourth ventricle of the brain, as observed by that justly-eminent physiologist. Brown Sequard. The specific gravity of urine was 1.037, and contained a considerable amount of sugar. Dr. Barlow and Sir William Gull have met with cases of Diabetes which have followed attacks of apoplexy, terminating in hemiplegia. The urine in these cases was of high specific gravity, and abundantly charged with sugar.

Diabetes has appeared in conjunction with softening of the base of the brain; with abscess in the cerebellum, extending into the fourth ventricle; with a tumour in the left lobe of the cerebellum; with diseases of the sympathetic nerve; with a tumour of the pneumogastric nerve; and with the deposit of bone in the falx major.

We have already referred to the experiments of M.M. Cyon and Aladoff, of St. Petersburg, who found that irritation of the annulas or valve of Vieussens produced white marks on the lobules of the liver, and gives rise to Diabetes. The vaso motor nerves of the artery are within the valve of Vieussens: division of these nerves causes the artery to dilate, and at the same time gives rise to Diabetes Mellitus.

Dr. Bichoff, Munich, says there is no disease where the diagnosis is so certain, but the pathology of which is hidden in such obscurity. Some attribute it to the nervous system; others to a change in the blood corpuscles. Dr. B. found fatty degeneration of the arteries of the brain a cause; likewise disease of the abdomen.

Diabetes Mellitus commits sad havoc amongst that class of men and women who put undue pressure upon the normal capabilities of the thinking principles of the brain, known as a fagged brain. For this reason it is of frequent occurrence among literary men, clergymen, arithmeticians, mathematicians, cashiers, and those who have embarked in the WEAR and TEAR, and constant anxiety, of a city or commercial life.

Diabetes has been known to follow sudden mental shocks, grief, or joy; and Rayer mentions a case in which the disease succeeded a violent paroxysm of rage. Prout refers the disease, in some instances, to the continued exposure to cold and moisture; to drinking cold fluids when the body is overheated; to the suppression of an habitual perspiration; and to a gouty or rheumatic diathesis. Sydenham and Senac, to violent horse exercise; Cheselden and Latham, to chronic abscesses and carbuncles; Frank, to the drying up of chronic eruptions, exanthems, leucorrhoea, or the suppression of haemorrhages; Boerhaave, to the abuse of diuretics and diluents; Autenreith, to acids and acidulous fluids; Ploucquet, to falls and injuries on the back, loins, and hips; and Bennewitz, in 1828, related the case of a female who was affected by the disease during two successive pregnancies. I have met with two cases which were clearly traceable to ovarian tumours. Latham mentions a case which was produced by the bite of a Rat; and Aretseus, as far back as A.D. 200, refers to the virus of a serpent, called Dipsas, occasioning Diabetes; and hence the common name given to the complaint in those days.

There are various other causes which do lead to a saccharine condition of the urine, and which may not inaptly come under the category of physical causes; the most notable being a passive congestion of the blood-vessels of one or more organs of the body. Claude Bernard, in his experiments on animals, clearly proved this. After obstructing the breathing of a dog for half an hour, to an extent short of causing death by asphyxia, the blood was found to present a strongly saccharine condition; whilst, previous to the experiment, it only contained the normal traces of sugar. This experiment was repeated on several other dogs, with a like result. In explanation of this effect, it may be said that by violent muscular efforts the liver will be compressed, and the escape of Glucogene from its cells promoted. During the existence of congestion, an unnatural relation between the contents of the cells and the blood-vessels will subsist, and changes may thus take place that would not otherwise occur. Besides this, the effect of detention of the blood in the vessels will be to compress the liver cells, and hasten the transudation of their contents. To give a practical and clinical illustration of this, we have simply to refer to two or three well-known diseases.

1. WHOOPING-COUGH.— The protracted paroxysms of coughing in this complaint, not only occasion a great amount of venous congestion — as clearly indicated by the dark and livid appearance of the countenance of the little patient — but the liver also, at the same time, must suffer from a considerable amount of compression, from the violent action of the inspiratory and expiratory muscles. Hence a saccharine condition of the urine is often observed.

2. PNEUMONIA.— Where a large mass of lung tissue becomes suddenly attacked by inflammation, great difficulty of breathing becomes a prominent symptom of the complaint. As a secondary consequence, there will be a proportionate obstruction to the free passage of blood through the lungs, more particularly when the inflammation has reached its second stage — that of hepatization. The liver in this case, also, will become necessarily implicated in common with the surrounding organs; and, as a result, a " saccharine" condition of the urine will be observed.

COMA. — A state of stupor, with loss of consciousness, from which the patient is roused with difficulty, being the consequence of the loss of nervous power, constitutes this alarming disease. The breathing becomes laboured, stertorous, and slow. An impediment here likewise to the flow of blood through the lungs is thus produced, and the liver, participating in the mischief, will be placed in a similar condition as to its glucogenic phenomena.

ASTHMA. — In the generality of cases of Asthma and Emphysema of the lungs, with its corresponding venous congestion of the liver, we shall have little difficulty in tracing a saccharine condition of the urine.

CHLOROFORM and ETHER. — Reynoso was about the first physiologist who pointed out that, after the inhalation of chloroform or ether, a certain amount of sugar was to be found in the urine. He attributed this phenomena to a diminished activity of the respiration, leading to a deficient oxidation of the sugar supposed to exist in the blood flowing through, the lungs. The intensity of the struggling and con« gestion that often ensues, may also have much to do with the intensity of the saccharine deposit.

CARBUNCLES and BOILS.— A saccharine condition of the urine has long been recognised as a frequent, if not an invariable associate of these very painful tumours. The relationship of the co-existence of these phenomena still remains a disputed point as to whether a Diabetic constitution engenders these boils and carbuncles, or whether they precede the characteristic symptoms of Diabetes.

BLOOD. — An altered — consequently abnormal — condition of the blood circulating through the liver may give rise to such a transformation of glucogenic substances into sugar, as to occasion a strongly saccharine state of the blood, and thence of the urine. It must, however, be observed, that a supply of portal blood is absolutely necessary for the glucogenic substance to be maintained in its normal state, and without undergoing transformation into sugar. There are, however, certain elements which, when admitted into the portal circulation, whether as medicines or otherwise, do undoubtedly exercise a deleterious influence over the normal glucogenic substances as found in the hepatic cells. Harley injected small quantities of ether and ammonia into the portal system: the result was a distinctly recognisable appearance of sugar in the urine. M. Leconte administered small doses of the nitrate of uranium, which was followed by similar results.

Pavy administered (by injection or otherwise, he does not say) phosphoric acid, which produced such a condition of the blood as to promote the transformation of glucogenic substances into sugar, to a sufficient extent as to give rise to strongly-marked glycosuria; and this condition appeared within one hour of the administration of the phosphoric acid.

Schiff has advanced the opinion, that it is to the development of a ferment in the blood that the production of Glucogene may be ascribed. He asserts that the blood of the living animal, under normal circumstances, is devoid of ferment capable of acting upon the glucogenic substance of the liver; and hence, he says, the escape of this principle from undergoing transformation during life.

Various lesions of the nervous system, by destroying the influence winch it exercises during life, under natural conditions, of holding in check the strong chemical tendency of glucogenic substance to undergo transformation into sugar, may also be considered as a cause of Diabetes Mellitus; the operations of this cause being well illustrated by the rapid production of sugar in the liver after death, and by the saccharine condition of the urine, induced by maintaining the circulation by artificial respiration for an hour or so, after the destruction of life, by pithing, by Woorali poison, and by strychnia; also by lesions of certain portions of the nervous system, especially of the medulla oblongata, which appears to exercise a marvellous influence over the circulation of the liver and the glucogenic substances, as proved by the experiments of Claude Bernard, Pavy, and others.

Dr. Donkin considers that Diabetes may possibly depend on a perverted functional action of the liver cells, whereby they morbidly secrete Diabetic sugar instead of Glucogene, their normal secretion. "This," says Donkin, "is a much simpler explanation of the nature of the disease; and it is, moreover, not at variance with our knowledge of the varied secreting power of gland-cells, or glandular epithelium, of which the liver-cells are a modification. For example, the secreting gland-cells of the mammary glands, during the period of lactation, secrete lactin, or milk sugar, which closely resembles Diabetic sugar; and this, too, in animals subsisting on food containing not a trace of starch or sugar. Thus we know that milk sugar is found in the milk of the carnivora, and of dogs fed exclusively for months on an animal diet. Judging from analogy, then, may not grape sugar be secreted by the glandular cells of the liver as an abnormal secretion in Diabetes? We could thus account for the appearance of functional activity which this organ frequently, if not generally, presents after death from the disease." — This opinion, however, is purely conjectural; but as the various theories hitherto propounded as to the exact cause of Diabetes are, to a great extent, more or less conjectural, the theory put forth by Dr. Donkin is worthy of more than a passing: thought.

Brain and Spinal Cord.— Dr. W. H. Dickinson, of London, endeavours to show that Diabetes is essentially an affection of the brain and spinal cord, and that the views hitherto entertained that Diabetes is a functional disorder, must be regarded as only provisional, inasmuch as function is simply an expression of structure; the two standing in relation to each other as cause and effect; and that where, as in Diabetes, the function is permanently altered, it almost follows, of necessity, that there should be equally abiding changes in the mechanism of the organs concerned. Acting in accordance with these views. Dr. Dickinson dissected the bodies of those who had died of Diabetes, and found that the brain and spinal cord were the seat of important structural alterations — a fact which gained more than ordinary significance from C. Bernard's brilliant discovery, that puncture of a particular part of the medulla oblongata produced a saccharine condition of the urine. His *"post-mortems"* revealed peculiar morbid changes in every part of the brain, medulla oblongata, and spinal cord; being most particularly marked in the medulla oblongata and pons varolii. There was dilatation of the arteries, and degeneration of the nervous matter external to them. And he further considers that these are not changes produced by the saccharine condition of the urine, but that they are antecedent to, and the original cause of, the Diabetes.

Notwithstanding the rapidly-increasing number of observations; the discovery of many obscure causes, or supposed causes; and the very close alliance which exists between the normal functions of the liver and Diabetes Mellitus — as pointed out to us in the brilliant and astounding experiments of Claude Bernard within the last twenty years — it is a matter of considerable astonishment to me, that so little is known of, and still less referred to, the anatomical lesions found in the hepatic structure in connection with a saccharine condition of the urine. English authorities, of a recent date, are more or less silent upon this point. Prout, Copland, Harley, and Donkin do not refer to it; and the only reference made to it by Pavy is embodied in the following few words: — " Morbid anatomy has contributed NOTHING towards elucidating the pathology of Diabetes. We refer the origin of the sugar encountered in the disease to a faulty action of the liver; but there is NO STRUCTURAL CHANGE OF the ORGAN to be discovered, as there is, for instance, in the case of the kidney under the existence of albuminuria. We have a manifestation of a disordered functional action to deal with without any discernible anatomical alteration to account for it." — Let us, however, see, as we think we shall be able to prove to the contrary a little further on. Mead, an eminent physician of the past century, was about the first to point out structural lesions of the liver in connection with Diabetes. This, years afterwards, was confirmed by Cawley and Hecker. Cullen, Franck, and Home, however, recognised no such alterations.

There is, however, a certain form of hypertrophy of the liver to be met with, which is undoubtedly very closely allied with Diabetes Mellitus. It is, however, a form of enlargement which has no relationship whatever with — consequently must not be confounded with — hydatids, fatty and waxy infiltrations, pyaemic or tropical abscess. The form of enlargement which I refer to, is that which presents a uniformity of contour, and exceeds in size two, three, or even four times its normal dimensions. It is accompanied by a simple increase in the size or the number of the secreting cells; and its consistence is at one time dense and firm, at another time soft and flabby; whilst the quantity of blood contained in its vessels may be increased or diminished.

Anatomically. — By hypertrophy of the liver, we understand an enlargement of that organ, with a proportionately enlarged size, or number of the secreting cells. Comparatively few traces can be discovered of the nutritive changes constantly occurring in the normal liver. Structural forms, indecisive, on the one hand, of the development or new formation of the glandular cells, or, on the other, of their disintegration, are so rarely met with, that one is forced to regard them as differing from the cells of other glands in being of a more persistent nature. Under certain circumstances, however, this condition undergoes a remarkable alteration; and changes make their appearance which are unquestionably indicative of an increased growth, or of a rapid new formation, of the elementary glandular structures: cells are observed in the enlarged organ, which attain two or three times the natural size; and each of these contains two or three large sharply-defined nuclei, each being provided with one or several vesicular nucleoli. These cells are easily separable from one another, and have an irregularly angular form: their contents are more or less granular, and occasionally include isolated oil-globules, or pigment granules. The lobules of the gland are enlarged to an extent corresponding to the growth of the cells, and stand out distinctly from the cut surface.

In other cases, we observe small, rounded, pale cells, firmly adherent to one another, with a large nucleus, and only slightly opaque cell-contents, and at the same time numerous free, round and oval, granular nuclei. When the small cells predominate, the outline of the lobules is not very distinct, and the cut surface of the organ is usually of a uniform reddish-brown colour; and the normal volume of the liver, as a natural consequence of this increase in the size and number of the cells, undergoes considerable enlargement.

The circumstances under which this increased growth or formation of the secreting cells of the liver takes place are numerous. Thus hypertrophy of the liver has been observed in cases where one portion of the organ has been destroyed by syphilitic inflammation, obliteration of the branches of the portal vein, or other exudation processes. It has been met with in cases of long persistent determination of an abnormal quantity of blood to the liver — Hyperaemia. This may take place in Asthma, Emphysema, Whooping-cough, Pneumonia, and Leukaemia; for, in addition to the enlargement of the spleen and lymphatic glands in patients suffering from that peculiar condition of the blood, the liver is found frequently to be considerably enlarged in Leukaemia.

There are certain forms of Diabetes Mellitus also in which this form of enlargement of the liver plays a very important part; and it will now become my duty to record a few interesting cases connected with this subject, chiefly collected by Frerichs.

In the winter of 1849, Frerichs examined, at Gottingen, the liver of a man, aged 44, who had died of Diabetes Mellitus, pulmonary tubercle, with pneumo-thorax. The liver was considerably enlarged; its form natural, and its outer surface smooth. Its connecting tissue — parenchyma — was much congested, and of a uniform brownish-red colour, without any distinct indication of lobules; its consistence was dense and firm. The cells were intimately adherent, and unusually pale; their form rounded, and their size varied from 1/200 to 1/120 of a line. All of them contained a large shining nucleus, and only a small quantity of grey, or, occasionally, yellowish granules. In addition to these cells, numerous rounded nuclei, with nucleoli, were observed, and also young cells, with the cell wall closely applied to the nucleus. This patient was a husbandman, and had been previously treated, at the Holtensen Academical Hospital, for Diabetes; ultimately terminating in tubercle, pneumo-thorax, and death. Eight days before death, the sugar disappeared from the urine; while the specific gravity, which had previously varied from 1.030 to 1.038, fell to 1.023, and ultimately to 1.010. The kidneys as well as liver were considerably enlarged, firm, and congested.

The second case was that of a woman, aged 37, who was treated for Diabetes Mellitus, and who died from caries of the petrous bone and erysipelas, in 1854, in the Clinique at Breslau. The same abnormalities were found in her liver.

In a third case of Diabetes Mellitus, which was treated in the Hospital of the Brothers of Charity at Breslau, similar *post-mortem* appearances were found in the liver of this person.

Stock vis, in 1856, examined the liver of a female, aged 30, who had died from Diabetes Mellitus: he found it considerably enlarged, and was able to trace the appearances indicative of an abnormal cell-growth — viz., large cells, some of which contained several nuclei, young cells, and free nuclei.

C. Bernard, in 1855, found the liver congested and considerably enlarged in the body of a Diabetic patient, who had died suddenly from pulmonary apoplexy; it weighed 88 1/10 oz. avoirdupoise, [1] and contained more than double the absolute quantity of sugar in a normal liver.

Hiller, in 1843, saw the liver and kidneys increased to three or four times their natural size, and the spleen double its normal size, in a man who had died of Diabetes Mellitus.

In a case of Diabetes Mellitus which occurred in my own practice five years ago — the subject a male, aged 55, and a near relative, the specific gravity of whose urine, when first tested, amounted to 1.050 — I found, on careful palpation, considerable enlargement of the liver, which, with the intense thirst, saccharine urine, and the other abnormal symptoms, entirely disappeared at the close of eight weeks' treatment, which consisted of Turkish baths, compresses to the hypochondrium, and the administration of Aconite, Leptandra, Podophyllum, and Nux Vomica, with a judiciously selected diet.

J. P., aged 52, consulted me in March, 1873, suffering from confirmed Diabetes of four months' standing; the specific gravity of his urine varied from 1.038 to 1.050. He was a generous liver, and partook freely of malt liquor: he suffered more or less from dyspepsia; the bowels were habitually costive. Careful palpation of the hypochondriac region revealed considerable enlargement of the liver. Turkish baths, a wet compress over the liver, and the administration of Aconite, Leptandra, Nux Vom., Merc. Sol., and Podophyllum, followed by Sulphur, sufficed to eradicate these symptoms in three months.

The Rev. T. L., a Welsh minister of the established church, consulted me in June, 1872 — chiefly afterwards by correspondence. He had suffered from Diabetes Mellitus for more than twelve months. The specific gravity of his urine, when first seen, ranged from 1.040 to 1.050, and held in solution a large quantity of saccharine matter. He was a large eater; and living in a somewhat remote part of the country, where fresh meat was a scarcity, he partook rather frequently of fat bacon and roof beef, with a too-liberal allowance of the national beverage — the nut-brown ale of the far-famed Vale of Llangollen, Careful inspection by palpation, revealed considerable uniform enlargement of the liver. He was submitted to a similar treatment to that prescribed in the two former cases, which entirely removed the disease within three months.

Dropsy. — General as well as local Anasarca is not an uncommon complication, particularly in the advanced stage of Diabetes Mellitus. I have met with five cases of the kind; and however strange it may appear, the inordinate flow of urine had not the slightest effect in checking the dropsical effusion.

Cataract. — Disorders of vision are of frequent occurrence in Diabetes, more especially a peculiar opacity of the crystalline lens, known as Cataract. This phenomena was first pointed out by Dr. Prout; and Mr. France has since shown that it is one of the secondary affections produced by a saccharine condition of the blood. Mitchell, Richardson, and Staeber are of opinion that Cataract, connected with Diabetes, is due to the direct action of the sugar on the crystalline lens. That such a condition will follow the introduction of sugar into the circulation, is beyond doubt, as Mitchell and Richardson have proved this by injecting simple syrup beneath the skin of a frog, and in twenty-four hours the lens had become perfectly opaque. To effectually produce this phenomena, the specific gravity of the syrup must exceed 1.045, or that of the blood.

Finally, whatever may be the immediate exciting cause of Diabetes, clinical history very clearly points to an hereditary constitutional peculiarity; for not only is it occasionally met with in more than one member of the same family, but it has even been found present in parent and child to the third generation. Dr. Mosler relates the case of a patient whose father, mother, two sisters, and a brother, died of Diabetes. Dr. Prout has observed it in four instances. Isenflamm states that he knew of seven of the descendants of a Diabetic patient who died of the malady. Brisbane, Rollo, Clarke, and others, furnish similar instances.

Pavy quotes a series of cases of a similar type, viz.: —

A Huddersfield gentleman, aged sixty-eight, who belongs to a family of seven, three of whom, besides himself, have been affected with Diabetes.

A gentleman, only twenty-three years old, who died of the complaint, had a father and aunt who succumbed to the same disease.

A former solicitor to the Treasury, with four near relatives, died from the same complaint.

A gentleman, aged sixty years, and a son only twenty-three years old, died of the same complaint.

Two brothers, clergymen, are attacked with the same disease.

Three brothers are affected with Diabetes; two die, the third still lives.

A lad, only thirteen years old, was under Pavy, at Guy's Hospital, in 1864; shortly after this he dies, when a sister, only nine years old, becomes similarly affected.

A gentleman writes me in March last, from Southport, relative to his brother, aged thirty-six, who is suffering from Diabetes, and concludes by stating that their mother died from the same disease.

Diabetes is more frequently met with in the male than in the female sex, and in persons who are either past the period of puberty, or are advanced in years. The true Diabetes Mellitus is rare in children; whilst albuminous urine, enuresis, or Diabetes Insipidus, are common complaints in them.

Diabetes is a disease of indefinite duration, the ordinary career being from two to three, and in exceptional cases its duration has reached ten, years.

The grave and fatal character of the disease in early life is well illustrated by Prout, who states that, in his extensive experience of forty years, and embracing nearly 700 cases, he witnessed twelve instances of Diabetes in young subjects between the ages of eight and twenty years, not one of whom reached the age of maturity; the majority dying in various ways, after a short course of the disease. Professor Christison, of Edinburgh, confirms these views. Griesinger, in an analysis of 225 cases, gives from two to three years as the average duration of the malady.

The incipient, or first stage of Diabetes, is the most protracted; and, according to Dr. Prout, may extend over two or three years. Graves, of Dublin, had a patie;at of this kind, who passed eighteen pints of urine daily, which held more than a pound and a-quarter of solid matter, chiefly saccharine matter.

The second stage is much more rapid in its progress; and if not held in constant check by careful diet and judiciously selected medicines, death generally closes the scene in a few months, and in some cases in a few weeks, from its first invasion. It is during this second, or advanced stage, that the various complications set in — viz., lung disease, carbuncle, furuncle, and gangrene, by which the further progress of the malady is so frequently cut short. And when not thus terminated, death sets in from extreme emaciation, exhaustion, and profound Coma.

Seeing, then, that this alarming and hitherto considered mysterious and intractable disorder, springing as it were from a multitude of equally mysterious and deeply-seated causes — causes many of which have, until the last few years, layed concealed in the very centre of the citadel of the nervous system, the tabernacle of the soul and its thinking principle — the knowledge and removal of which has baffled the skill and astuteness of the most learned physicians, from the classic and philosophic age of ancient Greece to the more practical, physiological, and pathological period of this the 19th century; — in taking a practical and purely clinical view of Diabetes Mellitus, we must trace to the fountain-head its pathological phases. — A saccharine condition of the uriije, its inordinate quantity and high specific gravity, stands only in the same relationship to the pathological phenomena of the disease, as the yellow tint of skin and conjunctiva does to a diseased liver; the bronzed countenance to disease of the supra-renal capsules; or the albuminous urine, with its anasarca and ascites, does to Bright's disease of the kidneys. They are, in fact, simply signs or outward manifestations of a corresponding inward disorganisation. It is the plaintive voice of suffering nature appealing to the physician for relief. We can, therefore, easily understand how a variety of morbid actions, quite distinct from each other, and perhaps of a diametrically opposite character, may produce such a train of morbid phenomena. Let us, by way of example, point out, that if the natural stimulus of the liver be exalted, an unnatural amount of saccharine matter will be secreted; and if the quantity formed be greater than the amount requisite to supply the wear and tear of the system, the superfluous quantity, which then acts towards the organism as a foreign body, will be sent out of the body with the urine; hence the disease, Diabetes Mellitus, is established. On the other hand, the case may be reversed, and there may still exist an abnormal amount of sugar in the blood, to be eliminated or passed off with the urine, notwithstanding that only the proper amount has been secreted by the liver. This must of necessity happen when, from any cause, the process of proper assimilation has been interfered with, and the body, from some defect in its normal functions, fails to consume its usual quantity of sugar.

Hence it is clear that we have two distinct forms of the same disease to grapple with — one which may aptly receive the name Diabetes from excessive formation of sugar; the other. Diabetes from defective assimilation of the saccharine matter, or malnutrition. Hence also two different modes of treatment, more particularly in the dietetic department.

Pavy and Harley also believe in two distinct types of Diabetes Mellitus. In one form, they are of opinion that the only error existing is a want of proper assimilative power over sugar: this occurs chiefly amongst old people. In the other form of the disease — which includes the majority of cases — it occurs most frequently in young subjects, and in those below the middle period of life; and there must exist, thinks Pavy, something additional to the want of assimilative power over sugar, inasmuch as the urine continues to be saccharine even when starch and sugar are carefully excluded from the food. Donkin, however, does not agree with the theory propounded by Pavy and Harley as to the two distinct types of Diabetes, but rather considers them as merely different stages of one and the same morbid process. The unnatural conditions which lead to the transformation of Glucogene into sugar — viz., a congested condition of the blood-vessels of the liver, a change in the quality of the blood, and the various lesions of the nervous system — have already been referred to. We will now proceed to discuss the last section connected with this interesting subject — namely, its treatment, therapeutic, dietetic, hygienic, and hydropathic.

[1] The average weight of a healthy liver is estimated at about 45 ounces.

Chapter Eight - Treatment of Diabetes

HAVING now disposed of the main features connected with the history, chemistry, anatomy, physiology, and pathology of Diabetes Mellitus, one more section of our discourse remains to be discussed — namely, its treatment.

A disease, the origin and cause of which has been so little known, and hidden in so much obscurity, has naturally taxed the energies of the medical profession in all ages; hence the vast array of various medicines which have been prescribed for the cure of this complaint. And if the causes, or, at all events, the supposed causes, of a saccharine condition of the urine have been numerous, the remedies, whether rational, empirical, specific, or expectant, have been trebly so: in fact, their name and number are legion. The means of cure employed in this disease (says Copland), have been varied exceedingly, according to the opinions entertained respecting its nature. Many remedies have also been resorted to, empirically, with reference either to their mode of operation, or to the presumed pathology of the malady. Like all intractable maladies (says Harley), Diabetes has had a great many " specifics " proposed for its treatment; and this is not surprising, seeing that the number of specifics generally increase in exact proportion to the irremediable character of the disease to cure. "The object," says Pavy, "to be attained in the treatment of Diabetes, is to control the elimination of sugar; and according to the extent that this can be effected, the symptoms of the disease are subdued. To effect this, there are two plans which should be put into practice at the same time; namely, careful dieting and drugs. Various medicinal agents have, from time to time, been recommended, chiefly suggested by the theory that has happened to be entertained, at the time, regarding the nature of the disease." — "The first and chief point," says Prout, "to be attended to in the treatment of Diabetes, is a carefully-selected diet." This is fully endorsed by most authorities of the present day.

"To write a history of the medicinal treatment of Diabetes," says Donkin, "would be an equally laborious and fruitless undertaking, inasmuch as almost every known medicine has been tried in succession, without the discovery, amongst them, of a single agent possessing a specific or curative action over the disease." But although it is not our intention to write an elaborate essay on this branch of the subject, nevertheless a brief sketch is fairly called for, were it only to point out to the reader the utter uselessness of treating diseases simply by their outward manifestations, and in total darkness and ignorance of their pathological phenomena.

Aretseus the Cappadocian, and contemporary of Gralen, A.D. 200, recommended cataplasms and ointments externally, which were made of nard, mastich, dates, raw quinces, and rose-oil, with the juice of acacia and hypocistis. If for ointment, these ingredients were mixed with wax and nard [1] ointment; if for a lotion, with water. But the water used as drink (says the same author), is to be boiled with autumn leaves. The food is to be milk; and with it the cereals, starch, groats, of spelt (alica), gruels. Astringent wines, to give tone to the stomach; and these but little diluted, in order to dissipate and clear away the other)mmours; for thirst is engendered by saltish things. But wine, which is at the same time astringent and cooling, proves beneficial, by inducing a change and good temperament; for to impart strength, sweet witie is like blood, which also it forms. The compound medicines are the same as that from vipers, the Mithridate, [2] that from autumn fruit, and the others which are useful in dropsy. But the whole regimen and course of life is the same. — Paulus Aegineta recommended plenty of good food difficult of digestion, and not humid; such as alica, with rose-wine, or rhodomel, or hydromel, or some wine that is not old, or some of the hot wines. He gave pot-herbs, succory, endive, and lettuces; of fishes, those that abide in the rocks; the feet and womb of swine; pears, apples, and pomegranates; and cold water to drink. They were to drink "propomata," from the juice of knotgrass, and elicampane in dark-coloured wine, and from the decoction of dates and myrtles. Cataplasms were applied to the hypochondrium and kidneys, of polenta in vinegar and rose oil, and of the leaves of the vine and navel-wort, pellitory of the wall, and purslain. He promoted sweats and vomiting by drinking cold water, and made them abstain from all sorts of diuretics. He also recommended bloodletting.

Both mineral and vegetable astringents have been recommended by many writers. Nitric acid, hydrochloric acid, sulphuric and the nitro-hydrochloric acid, either alone or combined with Cinchona, by Gilby, Brera, and Copland: sumach, kino, and catechu, by Willis, Fothergill, and Sydenham; phosphoric acid, phosphate of soda, and phosphate of iron by Sharkey and Venables: sulphate of zinc, sulphate of quinine, sulphate of alumina, sulphate of iron, and the super-sulphate of potash, by Wintringham, Frank, and Fraser: lime-water, milk. Cinchona, elixir of vitriol, simarouba, cascarilla, and the various preparations of iron, by Morton, Frank, and Steelier: Dover's powder. Opium, Camphor, antimonials, with the vapour and sulphur baths, by McCormick, Marsh, Eitter, and others: emetics, purgatives, and laxatives, by Rollo, Bichter, and Watt: Sulphur, the alkaline sulphurets, Cantharides, Valerian, Assafoetida, Myrrh, Cuprum Ammoniatum, and Tartar-emetic, by Autenreith,Bang, Werner, and Morgan: mercurial inunction, and the nitro-hydrochloric acid lotion applied over the hypochondria, by Lubbock and Scott: Calomel, Rhubarb, and Colchicum, by Brera and Frank: bleeding, leeches, blisters, setons, issues, and moxas, have been recommended from the age of Aetius down to Prout, Hufeland, Sir David Barry, and Watt: and stimulating liniments, composed of Camphor, Turpentine, soap. Capsicum, and oil of lemons, by Copland and others. My late friend. Dr. T. H. Tanner, in his Index of diseases, gives the following formidable array of medicines for Diabetes: — Opium, 1/2 to 1 grain, thrice daily; Codia, Opium, Ipecac, and Nitre, in a mixture; Citrate of Ammonia, or potash, with steel; reduced Iron, Aloes, and Nux Vomica, Strychnia, Quinine, and Opium; Kreasote, Cod-liver oil, or suet boiled in milk; peroxide of hydrogen; oxygenated water, Pepsine, Castor-oil; Seidlitz powders; compound powder of Rhubarb and Magnesia; aperient enemata; Carbonate of Soda; Acetate of Potash; Tartrate of Potash and Soda; Carbonate of Ammonia; Indian hemp; Permanganate of Potash, Alum, limewater, yeast, large quantities of sugar, potato-bread. Iodine, Nitric Acid, Phosphoric Acid, Sulphur, Turpentine, Permanganate of Potash, and inhalation of oxygen gas.

Copland, more than forty years ago, laid down a code of rules, which were adopted more or less by Parr and Prout, two great authorities at that period, who considered that the disease should be viewed in a twofold light. — First-ly, as respects its saccharine condition, independently of the increase of its quantity.

Secondly, as regards this state in connection with an augmented secretion, which should always be kept prominently in view: and although the dis-charge of an increased quantity of urine, in addition to its saccharine condi-tion, generally indicates either a more advanced or a more severe stage of the disease, yet we should be aware that the saccharine change is by far the most important of the two; and that it is much more easy to diminish the quantity than to improve the quality of this abnormal secretion. Copland ex-pressed great doubt — with whom Parr and Prout agreed — that there exist-ed a special drug capable of improving the condition of the urine; or at all events he knew of none. Such improvements can therefore be attempted only by those agents that tend to restore the general health and assimilative ener-gies of the frame, and to diminish the quantity of the secretion. To obtain these objects, we should endeavour to remove the congested, loaded, or op-pressed condition of the vascular system, and reduce the quantity of the cir-culating fluid more nearly to a level with the amount of vital power and as-similative function. — 2. To promote and improve the secretions employed in digestion, and excite the exhalations and secretions from the respiratory and intestinal surfaces.

3. To remove the unperspirable and harsh state of the cutaneous surface, to increase perspiration, and thereby to lessen the determination to the kid-neys.

4. To diminish the morbid sensibility and irritability of the frame, with the other morbid phenomena allied to them.

To promote these objects, Copland prescribed general and local blood-letting, followed by drastic purgatives, such as Colocynth and Turpentine; and when debility existed, the various preparations of iron or bark. The diet and regimen should be chiefly animal, with a small proportion of farinaceous substances; and the drink should consist of distilled water, lime-water and milk combined, alum, whey, and the Bristol hot-wells, or the Bath waters, or weak solutions of nitric or hydrochloric acid, boracic acid, or the subborate of soda.

Such is a brief outline of the remedies selected and the mode of treatment adopted by a large section of the leading Allopathic physicians for the last half century: but from the wonderful advances which have been made within the last twenty years, as to a more correct knowledge of the causes and pathological phenomena of this disease — thanks to the eminently scientific labours of Claude Bernard and others — the treatment has become proportionately more simple and rational, and the result more efficacious and successful.

Pavy — a no mean authority — confines his treatment to diet, mineral waters, opium, and one of its manifold properties — codia; with the acetate, citrate, and tartrate of potash, and soda.

Harley — to diet, hydrocyanic acid, strychnine, phosphoric acid, iron, bromide of iron, and opium.

Donkin — chiefly to skim-milk, which has been raised. " phoenix-like," from the ashes of Aretaeus, who prescribed it for Diabetes, A.D. 200. The rules laid down by Donkin are as follows: —

The skim-milk must be prescribed in carefully measured quantities. It must be given alone, and every other article of food must be strictly prohibited.

If a patient has an aversion for milk, or if he suffers from indigestion, or a feebled condition of the digestive organs, we must begin with small and well-regulated doses.

During the first day of the treatment, half a teacupful of skim-milk may be given every two or three hours; and on the second day, double the quantity at the same intervals; on the third day, half a pint may be allowed for each dose, and the intervals increased to three or four hours; so that, in all, three pints are consumed. On the fourth day, four pints may be given; on the fifth or sixth, five pints: and should this augmented quantity produce no inconvenience, and the patient's appetite is good — as it generally is under the treatment — the quantity may be raised to six or seven pints daily: but after this, no further increase should be permitted, except in certain cases of Diabetes in patients of large frame and keen appetites, to whom eight, or even nine pints may be allowed daily.

A limitation of the daily allowance of skim-milk to the quantity just stated, is of paramount importance in obtaining a successful issue of the case under treatment; consequently, six or seven pints should never be exceeded without some important reason.

So soon as the patient can digest the full daily allowance of skim-milk without inconvenience, it may be given at four separate meals, with an interval of four hours between each, or at shorter periods, and in a smaller quantity at a time. The milk may be given cold or warm, according to the inclination of the patient; but it must never be *boiled,* as a temperature of 212° seriously impairs, or altogether destroys its therapeutic energy, possibly by altering the molecular constitution of the caseine, or by destroying some vital property with which it is endowed.

The curative influence of skim-milk over Diabetes, may, Donkin thinks, be referred to two causes.

First, to the facility with which, by the processes of digestion and sanguification, it is transformed into healthy blood, which seems to have the power of regulating or controlling a healthy, and of preventing a diseased nutrition, in accordance with physiological laws.

Secondly, to the absence of all substances foreign to healthy nutrition; and which, when imported into the blood with the food, becomes a *materies morbi,* or the appropriate sustenance of morbid action or disease.

Dr. Devergir (*"La France Médicale,"* March 19th, 1876) observes, that cases of Diabetes differ extremely, and cannot all be treated alike. The cutting off of starchy diet is excellent; but it is a painful treatment in many cases, and many patients are apt to relax much in attention to its exigencies.

The privation of bread is kept to with great difficulty. He affirms that arsenical preparations have the power, in many instances, of getting rid of sugar from the urine. Called to treat a case of prurigo vulva in a lady, Dr. Devergir prescribed Arsenic; and it was soon discovered that the lady had glycosuria, in addition to prurigo. This lady was cured of both maladies by means of the employment of Arsenic. He then had the idea of treating all his Diabetic patients with Arsenic, and found the sugar often disappear completely, or become greatly lessened in quantity, without the patients much altering the diet.

Professor Cantini places great reliance on albuminous and other food, which do not minister to the production of sugar. He thus confines the sufferer to a regimen of fish, or other marine productions - "frutte di mare," as Italians term them — flesh-meat and plain water, or acidulated with lactic acid.

PHENIC ACID. —A complete cure of Diabetes Mellitus is related in the *"Bahia Medical Gazette,"* by means of phenic acid: two and a-half grains night and morning, in mint-water. The patient, a teacher of music, had been struck from his saddle by a falling tree. Trommer's test had shown a very large amount of glucose, or grape sugar, in the urine.

CITRATE OF SODA.— The "*Clinic*," August, 1876, copies, from the " *Medical Brief,*" a recommendation by M. Guyot Darmecy, of citrate of soda in the treatment of Diabetes, given in daily doses of half a drachm to one drachm. Analysis has shown that sugar disappears from the urine when this salt is used with the food, instead of common salt. And the researches of Woehler have indicated, that the alkaline salts of organic acid, when given in doses too small to produce purgative effect, are absorbed, and, their acid being burnt up in the respiratory process, they are eliminated by the urine as carbonates. Citrate of soda may thus place the system under the influence of an alkaline carbonate, which is indispensable to the interstitial combustion of the glucose of the food.

A very novel and simple mode of treating Diabetes has been recorded by Dr. Charteris, of the Glasgow Royal Infirmary, to which the motto, "shut your mouth and save your life," has received a new application. Coming in contact with an elderly and confirmed Diabetic in the Glasgow Infirmary, he received the following explanation of his own treatment, who discovered it after this wise. He found that he commenced to wheeze when he breathed the cold air, and that it ceased on his return to a warm room. On putting his head below the bed-clothes, a slight perspiration came upon him; the saliva returned, and his tongue and mouth became moist instead of dry, as formerly. When he withdrew his head again, and breathed in the open, his mouth and tongue again became dry and parched. This moistness and dryness of the mouth, alternately occurring under the conditions mentioned, having arrested his attention, the question arose in his mind — How could this moisture be obtained without remaining in bed? To accomplish this, he put on a respirator, and also a knitted woollen cloth over both the respirator and his nostrils when in the house, or even in bed, and was careful in protecting the nostrils as well when he' went out. He also began to practise breathing by the nostrils alone, and found that breathing exclusively in this manner, day and night, except when engaged in conversation, was highly beneficial. Having perfected himself in respiring by the nostrils alone, he laid aside both the respirator and the cloth, only muffling himself carefully up when he went out at night, or in frosty weather. He avoided going out at night as much as possible, and refrained from all cold diet and drink, invariably taking them warm. Under this treatment an amendment was apparent in less than fourteen days; and in less than a month it was very marked. This patient now lives like any other temperate man; and, being a very intelligent person, has formed his own theory in regard to the treatment. Briefly expressed in his own words, it is this — " Hitherto the attempt has been made to prevent production of sugar by giving a non-saccharine diet. This is, no doubt, perfectly correct; but in addition to this, the treatment I adopted was intended to promote the consumption of sugar produced. This design of consuming sugar by breathing through the nostrils in warm weather, or by means of a respirator, is, that when the proper quantity of sugar has been consumed, the abnormal production will then cease. The aim of this treatment is to raise the blood-heat to its proper temperature, and to restore to the lungs their partially-lost combustive power, and to enable them to consume as much secreted sugar as will remain in the blood at its proper temperature. When that purpose is accomplished, the organs will regain their proper function, and the patient recover."

Dr. Charteris has treated two cases of Diabetes in the Glasgow Royal Infirmary, and both have been much benefited.

[1] The spikenard of botanists.
[2] An ancient compound, having opium for its basis, and now replaced by the confection of opium.

Chapter Nine - Homoeopathic, Hydeopathic, Hygmenic, and Dietetic Treatment of Diabetes

THE Homoeopathic therapeutic agents of Diabetes Mellitus form a somewhat formidable array in number; but, like its Allopathically, but few have proved of any practical value. These I have arranged alphabetically, and are as follows: —

Aconitum Napellus, Acidum Nitricum, Acidum Hydrochloricum, Acidum Phosphoricum, Asclepias, Alumina, Ammonia Carb., Ambra Grrisea, Argentum Metallicum, Arnica Montana, Aurum Triphyllum, vel A. Maculatum, and Arsenicum Album.

Belladonna and Baryta Carbonica.

Cantharis, Carbo Vegetabilis, Cinchona, Chloral Hydrate, Clematis Erecta, and Conium.

Digitalis Purpurea.

Euphorbium Officinarum.

Grraphites.

Helonin.

Kali Carbonicum, Kreasote.

Magnesia Carbonica.

Mercurius Solubilis.

Muriate of Quinine.

Natrum Muriaticum.

Nux Vomica.

Plumbum Metallicum, Podophyllum Peltatum.

Saljcilic Acid, Strychnine, Sulphur, and Staphysagria.

Terebinthine.

Uranium Nitrate, and

Yeratrum Album.

We have here forty-one medicines, from which a selection has been made by different writers, as follows: —

Hempel selects Aconite, (p; Ars., 3 to 12; Merc. Sol., 3 to 6; Nux Yom., Ac. Nit., Acid. Phos., Arg. Met., Canth., Kreasote, and Squill. — See " Materia Medica."

Pulte. — Acid. Phosph., Carbo Veg., Conium, Merc. Sol., and Sulph. — See " Domestic Practice."

Laurie. — 1. Acid. Phosph., Merc. Sol., Sulph., Natrum Mur., Carbo Veg., and Ledum Palustre. 2. Acid. Hydrochlorid., Asclepias Vincetoxicum, Ammo. Carb., Arsenicum, Alumina, Grraphites, Ambra Grisea, Baryta Carb., Belladonna, Conium, Magnesia Carb., Terebinthine, Mephitis Putorius. Of these, says Laurie, the following have as yet been principally employed: — Merc. Sol., Verat., Kali Carb., and Acid. Hydroc. — See " Elements of Homoeopathic Practice."

Small. — Kali Carb., Acid. Hydroc, Merc. Sol., Staphysagria, and Veratrum Alb. — See Small's " Domestic."

Kuddock. — Acid. Phosph., Uranium Nitrate, Terebinthine, Aurum Triphyllum, Helonias, Muriate of Quinine, and Plumbum Met.; also Arsenicum, Digitalis, Nux Vom., Canth., Euphorbium Officinarum, China., and Merc, Sol.— See Kuddock's "Vade Mecum."

Bryant. — Arnica Montana, Argent. Met., Belladonna, and Phos. Acid. — Bryant's " Pocket Manual."

Becker, E. C. — Merc. Sol., Verat. Alb., and Kali Carb.; also Squilli, Carbo Veg., Causticum, Ledum Palustre, and Natrum Muriat. — See "American Homoeopathic Examiner."

Jahr, — Clematis Erecta. — See " Materia Medica."

Morgan (myself). — Aconite, Iris Versicolor, Leptandra, Nux Vomica, Podophyllum Peltatum, and Strychnine, in certain forms of the disease.

Let us now briefly review the pathogenesis of this imposing array of medicines, and see how far we should be justified in recommending them in a practical point of view.

ACONITE. — This valuable medicine is endowed with the power of deranging or embarrassing the capillaries of the liver, so far as to terminate in jaundice. If the portal capillaries are engorged to an extent as to interfere with their normal functions. Aconite relieves it. Aconite has a marked effect on acute, sub-acute, and even the chronic form of hepatitis. Aconite wonderfully controls congestion of the bowels, the lungs, heart, liver, and the whole of the pyloric region. Aconite covers a host of congestions of the cerebrospinal group. From these facts, we are justified in anticipating the most brilliant results to follow the administration of Aconite, in those cases of Diabetes which result from simple hypertrophy and hypersemia, with a perverted functional action of the liver-cells, whereby they morbidly secrete Diabetic sugar instead of Glucogene. It should be administered in the matrix form — one or two drops in pure water, and repeated every three or four hours.

ACID. NIT. diminishes the secretion of urine,, and moderates the thirst and heat in Diabetes. The most suitable potency is from the second to the sixth.

ACID. HYDROC. acts very similarly to Ac. Nit. It causes a frequent desire to urinate in health; consequently acts curatively in Diabetes.

ACID. PHOSPH. causes a frequent desire to micturate, the urine being either watery or cloudy. It should be selected for those cases of Diabetes where fatty degeneration of the liver, spleen, or kidneys, are suspected; with an albuminous as well as a saccharine condition of the urine; in impotency; in nervous depression; and in those cases arising from an abnormal condition in the nervous centres. Phosphorus, if administered in potent doses, causes a saccharine condition of the urine: it is, therefore a striking similar to the essential symptom of the disease. The potency should vary from the first to the sixth.

Dr. Holland, of Bath, records a case of Diabetes in a female, aged forty-four, the specific gravity of whose urine, when first seen, was 1.048, and the quantity of water passed in the twenty-four hours, over four quarts. She was cured, in four months, by Phos. Acid, and the Nitrate of Uranium.

Dr. Mary Walker has cured a case of Diabetes with a high dilution of Acid. Phos., and a nutritious diet; no food being exempt except potatoes.

"It is in Diabetes," says Richard Hughes, "that Phosphoric Acid has won its greenest laurels. Not only in the INSIPID form — 'chronic diuresis,' as we should now call it — but in true glycosuria, cure has repeatedly resulted from the administration of this acid. It is actually a similar to the essential symptom of the disease: for Dr. Pavy found saccharine urine to result from its injection into the general venous system, or introduction into the intestinal canal; and Griesinger, who gave it in Diabetes to the extent of an ounce a day, found the sugar increased thereby. But the frequent origin of Diabetes in the nervous centres (as suggested by Claude Bernard's well-known experiment), commends it still more forcibly; and in the only case in which I have myself needed it, to reinforce the Nitrate of Uranium, the disease obviously began in this way. It will therefore be in Diabetes of nervous origin that we shall expect to get the best results from Phosphoric Acid. Moreover, since Claude Bernard found Albuminuria to result from a central nervous lesion, hardby that which occasions Diabetes, there may well be cases of this malady in which Phosphoric Acid is indicated." Dose, several drops of the 1st decimal dilution.

ASCLEPIAS SYEIACA (Milk-weed) acts specifically on the urinary organs, either on the diminished or increased secretion.

ALUMINA points to a frequent desire to make water; an increased secretion of aqueous urine, with, at times, a white flocky deposit — albumenoids.

AMMONIUM CARBONICUM.— Several copious emissions of urine at night; frequent and copious emissions of a pale-yellow urine during night and day; continued thirst; a good deal of hunger and thirst.

AMBEA GRISEA. — An increased secretion of urine, with inability to retain it, in the morning; dryness of the mouth, tongue, and lips, early in the morning, when waking.

ARGENTUM METALLICUM.— A feeling of dryness in the tongue; violent appetite, even when the stomach is replete; excessive gnawing hunger the whole day, which cannot be satisfied by eating; frequent urging to urinate, with copious emissions of pale urine. Guided by these symptoms, Trinks recommended it in certain forms of Diabetes.

ARNICA MONTANA causes dryness in the mouth, with considerable thirst; a frequent desire to urinate, with a copious emission of pale urine; deglutition is prevented from an inordinate dryness of the mouth. Diabetes has been known to follow a blow on the liver. The Arnica, in such a case, would be a suitable remedy.

AURUM TRIPHYLLUM, vel MACULATUM (Wake-robin). — A greatly increased secretion of urine, which is watery and light-coloured, and smelling almost like burnt horn, with a slight cloud in the middle after standing.

The late Mr. W. Freeman, of Cardiff, South Wales, found this medicine to reduce the specific gravity of Diabetic urine from 1.038 to 1.028. The same authority noticed considerable enlargement of the *papillae circumvallatae* of the tongue in three cases of Diabetes Mellitus, with a peculiarly disagreeable taste at the back of the mouth at the same time.

Query. — Is the swelling of the *papillae circumvallatae* at all a constant sign of Diabetes? Does the Aurum Triphyllum produce the same abnormal conditions constantly? And, thirdly, does this drug at once, or after continued use, produce a saccharine condition of the urine?

ARENICUM ALBUM.— The physiologico-therapeutical range of Arsenic is only rivalled by the wonderful health-disturbing, and, therefore, health-restoring properties of Aconite. To the careful observer, the symptomatic resemblances of Aconite and Arsenic are remarkably striking. The various phenomena which Aconite seems to play on the surface of the organic functions, is performed by Arsenic in the very inmost recesses of vitality. The Aconite fever, for instance, is evanescent — a chill, or some slight chilly creepings or shiverings along the back, followed by a moderate degree of heat and moisture, corresponding in quality with the intensity of the previous rise of temperature.

The arsenical chill, on the contrary, seems to chill the vital blood in the very laboratory of the heart; and the subsequent heat is like a consuming fire burning up the vital moisture of the skin-pores, until a soaking, debilitating perspiration is supplied by the reactive forces of the living organism, as a restorer of their disturbed harmony.

We may further mention typhoid fever as another lesion strikingly illustrative of the difference of action between Aconite and Arsenic. Either of these agents may be adapted to a pathological lesion, which we designate as typhoid fever.

And yet how much more intensely is the vitality of the organism prostrated in typhoid, for which Arsenic is required, than in the same typhoid fever which may be controlled with Aconite. The later form of typhoid fever may not seem much worse than a severe attack of influenza, with mild exacerbations of fever every evening or afternoon, which are followed by more or less perspirations. But the type of typhoid fever to which the Arsenic is Homoeopathic, would be much more prominently marked: the chill is more racking, the subsequent fever-heat more burning, and the perspiration more debilitating. The vital fluids are much more deeply affected by the morbid process; the signs of decomposition more evident; there is a more manifest tendency to the formation of sores and petechiae; the bowels are either more tympanitic and torpid; or else the diarrhoea is more offensive and prostrating. In the Arsenic typhoid also, the urine is dark brown, foul, and scanty. In the Aconite form of the same fever, the urine may simply have a deep colour, and some sediment, without the quantity being altered.

We may draw a similar parallel in every disease to "which both Aconite and Arsenic are Homoeopathic.

Take a case of Asiatic cholera. In its mild form the symptoms will yield kindly enough to Aconite; but in the severe form, when the very mainsprings of life are invaded, paralysed, and strangled by that subtle poison, then Arsenic would have to be administered in fairly potent doses. Arsenic is one of those powerful medicines, that it penetrates into the inmost recesses of organic life, and poisons the very emanations of vitality as they diffuse themselves throughout the tissues. It is upon these grounds that Arsenic constitutes a formidable opponent to general debility: marasmus; wasting away of the fatty tissue; atrophia nervosa; atrophy of the spinal marrow; atrophy of the mesenteric glands in children; the marasmus of drunkards; gangrene of the various organs and extremities of the body; malignant pustules; boils and carbuncles; icterus senilis; cirrhosis; fatty degeneration, and tubercles of the liver. Consequently, Arsenic ought to play a very important part, as a curative and palliative agent, in prolonged and the more advanced stage of Diabetes Mellitus, and its grave complications.

In Diabetes Mellitus, *Arsenic* is, to a great extent, indicated by the symptoms. It is, however, problematical whether its Homoeopathicity extends to the essential character of the pathological process that is going on in the organism — at all events, in all cases. However, let us see. The process of nutrition in this disease is markedly defective in a specific direction. The nutritive principles which should repair the waste of tissues are abnormally eliminated by the kidneys as saccharine matter. The carbo-hydrates — of which sugar is one — do not constitute the basis of tissue; but sugar is a most important agent in the metamorphosis of animal matter. It is believed that the sugar which is found in the liver, owes its origin to the decomposition of albumenates, and more especially to fibrine. This fact, which was first discovered by Claude Bernard, and afterwards by Frerisch, has since been fully substantiated by numerous analyses, made by Lehmann, of the blood of both the portal and hepatic veins. Lehmann likewise suggests that the tendency of albumenates to pass into butyric fermentation — a tendency which is more particularly seen in the case of fibrine and caseine — may possibly be accounted for by the presence of a carbo-hydrate, sugar. Hence sugar, not only that which is introduced into the system in the form of starch, but also the Glucogene (sugar) which is manufactured in the liver, is essential to the process of assimilation.

The symptomatology and pathogenesy oi *Arsenicum Album* stamps it as a vehicle capable of striking down this process of mal-assimilation in its very onset. The action of Arsenic upon the system is characterised by all those symptoms which mark the morbid elimination of sugar by the urine. Hence we may fairly infer that most favourable results may follow the administration of Arsenic, in various potencies, in Diabetes Mellitus. It may go far to counteract that condition of the nervous system which permits the abnormally excessive formation of sugar in the organism, and the consequent deficiency in the re-production of the various tissues. It may go far, in conjunction with Phosphoric Acid, and other kindred remedies, to remove that tendency to fatty degeneration of the liver, and other organs of the body, found after death in certain forms of Diabetes Mellitus.

The conversion of bodies that had been poisoned by large quantities of Arsenic into adipocere, seems to show that that mineral must hold some specific relationship to the metamorphosis of animal tissues into fat. Lehmann has shown very conclusively that the fats are powerful auxiliaries in the formation of cells and tissues; and that, on the other hand, sugar is essential to the formation of adipose tissue. During the conversion of bodies into adipocere, every trace of Arsenic disappears. Is it, then, under such circumstances, irrational to suppose that Arsenic may be in specific relation with that inimical principle which, in the living organism, paralyses the assimilative nerve-force in a specific direction, and causes the abnormal elimination, in the form of sugar, of the primary principles essential to the process of reproduction?

Vogt claims for Arsenic a higher power to influence the metamorphosis of the tissues than is possessed by any vegetable drug extant. In this respect alone it far surpasses any of the other minerals in its peculiar penetrating power. This may seem more or less theoretical; but the long-continued effects of Arsenic upon the living tissues evince a power of disorganisation which no other agent can claim to the same extent. We may, therefore, rationally infer that this power may be made use of for the purpose of extinguishing, or neutralising, as it were, a pathological process, which results in such organic disorders as Arsenic is capable of producing.

Guided by the leading principle of our law, we have a just right to claim this power for Arsenic. It is, however, a misfortune, that the physical changes which large doses of drugs effect in the character of the urinary secretion, have not as yet been studied by positive experimentation, except in a limited number of cases; and on this account it is much to be regretted that the various " provers " of our remedies were not urged to test the urine for sugar in the course of their interesting experimental investigations, as it is more than probable that the urine, whilst under the influence of many drugs, would have yielded more than the normal quantity of saccharine matter. This, however, has been proved by Terebinthine, which shall be more particularly referred to when we come to discuss the pathogenesy of that medicine. Whether Arsenic will, under favourable circumstances, effect the abnormal elimination of sugar by the urine, remains to be determined by subsequent experimentations.

Barring this uncertainty. Arsenic covers all the constitutional symptoms which supervene in the course of Diabetes Mellitus.

Prominently among these, we notice —

1. An increased flow of urine.

2. A dry, brittle, and scaly condition of the skin.

3. A dryness of the mouth, fauces, tongue, and trachea, with an unquenchable thirst.

4. Loss of appetite.

5. Constipation.

Among the diagnostic symptoms of "Arsenical disease," we meet with a burning sensation, which extends from the coeliac plexus along the oesophagus, as far as the mouth, and the patient dwindles down to a mere skeleton; he loses strength, and sometimes his teeth. All these pathognomonic phenomena of Diabetes Mellitus likewise characterise the special action of Arsenic upon the various tissues of the body as well. Future observations, and more complete provings, may determine whether the urine, under the influence of Arsenic, will exhibit, those abnormal characters which go to constitute that fluid whilst under the ban of Diabetes Mellitus — namely, its tendency to become abnormal in quantity, of a sweetish taste, of a high specific gravity, of an opalescent or greenish tint, and the gradual disappearance of urea and uric acid. In the course of the provings of Arsenic by Hahnemann and others, it may be, that had the urine been tested for sugar, such would have been found. Be this, however, as it may. Arsenic has, and will still continue to play, an important part in the treatment of certain forms of Diabetes Mellitus, either alone or in alternation with Aconite and other carefully-selected remedies.

Hempel has treated successfully several cases of Diabetes Mellitus with Aconite, Merc. Sol., and Arsenicum, in potencies varying from the third to the twelfth dilution.

BELLADONNA is a medicine of potent agency; and seems to act primarily upon the cerebrospinal system of nerves, and to affect the vascular system secondarily. As an inflammatory-producing medicine, it stands on equal grounds with Aconite; but their primary and secondary action are the reverse of each other. Aconite, for instance, produces inflammation by depressing the functional power of the capillary ramifications of the ganglionic nerves, leaving the brain undisturbed, except in so far as it suffers from the effects of the functional derangement of any portion of the nervous system. BELLADONNA causes inflammation by first depressing the brain, after which the functional power of the ganglionic system becomes similarly, but secondarily, affected. Belladonna, consequently, acts precisely in a reverse order. It affects the brain primarily, and the ganglionic system incidentally: whereas Aconite affects primarily the ganglionic, and incidentally the brain.

The first effect of Belladonna upon the brain is to depress or unhinge its functional power; and, incidentally, the functional power of the ganglionic system. The stage of organic reaction is characterised, as in the case of Aconite, by capillary engorgements — viz., a full, rapid, and bounding pulse; glowing redness of the eyes; protrusion and suffusion of the eyes; heat of the skin, &c. But in the case of Belladonna, the antagonism seems to be between the capillaries and the central point of the nervous system, the brain: whereas, in the case of Aconite, the antagonism is between the capillaries and the terminal ramifications of the ganglionic system. Hence, in the case of Belladonna, the antagonism is marked by more obstinate, more deep-seated, and more dangerous symptoms than in the case of Aconite.

The inflammatory action of Belladonna may develop different forms of inflammation — viz., the simple, phlegmonous, erysipelatous, rheumatic, and gangrenous; and its Homoeopathicity ranges in a special manner over the various congestive and inflammatory conditions of the brain and its membranes — viz., meningitis, arachnoiditis, encephalitis, mania-apotu, myelitis, and that form of encephalitis induced by concussion of the brain; the result of a fall or blow; or from exposure to cold. It likewise covers apoplexy, paralysis, and certain forms of epilepsy.

Amongst the leading causes of Diabetes Mellitus, stands, prominently, certain injuries to the head, with or without fracture of the skull. These may follow falls, or blows on the back, top, or side of the head, resulting in concussion of the brain, or in the extravasation of blood; in meningitis, arachnoiditis, and phrenitis. For such a condition Belladonna is indispensable, and should be administered in potencies varying from the first to the third potency. When it may be found desirous to act freely on the skin, an alternating dose of Aconite should be given, or a series of Turkish baths.

BARYTA CARBONICA gives us as its symptoms— dryness of the tongue and mouth early in the morning, with a frequent emission of urine both by day and night.

CANTHARIS VESICATORIA. — The primary effect of Cantharis is to cause strangury; its secondary effect is that of a paralytic inability to retain the urine. This physiological fact suggests the use of Cantharides in both incontinence of urine and even Diabetes: it causes frequent and profuse micturition of a pale colour, and white flocculent sediment; hence Cantharis is suitable in cases of Diabetes complicated with Albuminuria, &c.

CARBO VEGETABILIS.— Both Pulte and Laurie record this substance as a remedy in Diabetes. Hahnemann gives the following pathogenetic effects: — Great dryness in the mouth early when waking; excessive thirst and hunger; pain in the liver, as if bruised; frequent desire to urinate, with anxiety day and night; *Diabetes;* general physical depression; great lassitude and languor after a short walk, with attacks of sudden weakness and fainting. The moral symptoms are striking: there is an indescribable anguish; oppression of the chest; general uneasiness, impatience, and great irritability.

CHINA, C. MURIATE OF QUININE.— Recent investigations tend to prove that Diabetes Mellitus is sometimes due to a diseased condition of the pancreas: at all events, fatty degeneration, dilatation, and atrophy of the spleen, are frequently found in those who have died of Diabetes. The well-known affinity which exists between Quinine and the spleen, points it out as a valuable remedy in cases of that kind. Even in cases where the patient has only had a mixed diet, small doses of the Muriate of Quinine have been found to remove the sugar from the urine.

CHLORAL HYDRATE.— A case is reported in the "Medical Times and Gazette," of the sudden Diabetic condition of the urine following the administration of Chloral Hydrate, given for sleeplessness. A dose of 20 grains (which failed to produce sleep) was followed by frequent micturition, producing, in the aggregate, 104 oz. of urine, of specific gravity 1.026. The abnormal condition gradually subsided after the use of the Chloral was discontinued. Chloral Hydrate, under such circumstances, may be selected as a curative agent in certain forms of Diabetes, particularly when connected with an over-wrought or fagged brain.

CLEMATIS ERECTA.— The provings of this drug are but obscure: there is frequent micturition, but little at a time. Hull's Jahr gives it a prominent note as a Diabetic remedy.

CONIUM. —Both Pulte and Laurie refer to Conium as a remedy in Diabetes.

In man, Conium seems to act primarily upon the brain, the cerebro-spinal, and the ganglionic systems of nerves. We have learnt from cases of poisoning that Conium causes apoplexy, paralysis, and epileptic seizures; consequently, Conium may be found very useful in cases of Diabetes arising from those abnormal conditions of the brain and its coverings. The pathogenetic effects, as applicable to Diabetes in general, are striking. They are marked by great exhaustion, faintishness, general languor of body and mind, lowness of spirits, and drowsiness; dryness and itching of the skin with petechiae; dryness of the tongue and mouth; aching or a painful lacerating in the liver; constipation; urgent desire to urinate every half -hour; Diabetes; Diabetes accompanied by great pain; frequent urging without stool; frequent urging every day, a small quantity only being expelled every day; impotence, cataract, opacity of the cornea, amaurosis, and presbyopia.

DIGITALIS. — This medicine may be expected to be of considerable service in cases of Diabetes occurring in the aged, subject to epileptiform seizures, general lassitude, vertigo, and intermittent pulse; emaciations of the body proportionate to an increase of intellectual activity; and the serous apoplexy of old age. Its pathogenesy yields a corrosive itching and peeling-off of the skin; an irregular, weak pulse; anxiousness, with great apprehension of the future; violent lancinating headache; amaurosis; objects appear either green or yellow; dryness of the throat; great thirst; costiveness; and a continual desire to pass water.

EUPATORIUM PERFOLIATUM.— This medicine stands upon a par with the various preparations of bark, and covers the different types of intermittent fever; consequently may be administered in those cases of Diabetes Mellitus connected with enlargement of the spleen, &c.

GRAPHITES. — This medicinal agent covers many of the symptoms of Diabetes, and would doubtless act beneficially in cases connected with a broken-down, gouty, and rheumatic constitution. It points to emaciation and general debility; twitching of the limbs; a paralytic sensation in all the joints; chronic dryness of the skin; itching of the skin; uneasy, sleepless nights; bleeding from the nose at night; dejection of spirits; want of disposition to work; continued forgetfulness; dryness of the mouth; hunger, and a constant craving for food; tightness, as from a firm band in the hypochondria; hard, knotty stools; frequent micturition, both by day and night; decrease of the sexual instinct; oppression of the chest; palpitation of the heart; general uneasiness of the limbs; boils, carbuncles, hepatic and scaly eruptions on the body.

HELONIAS DIOICA, in the l x trituration, cured a case of Diabetes in the hands of Hale and Paine, of Chicago, USA.

KALI CARBONICUM.— Both Laurie, Small, and the "North American Examiner," refer to this medicine as a remedy in Diabetes. The pathogenetic effects of this drug give us frequent weariness and depression of strength, dryness of the skin, and deficient perspiration; herpes, ascites, and anasarca; restless nights, great despondency, sadness, and irritability of temper; absence of mind; appetite depraved; a great desire for sleep during a meal; pain and pressure in the region of the liver; costiveness; frequent desire to urinate — the water pale and greenish; a deficient sexual instinct: no erections for three weeks and more.

KREASOTE. — Pereira observes that Kreasote increases the secretion of urine, but that in Diabetes Mellitus it decreases it. It may therefore prove efficacious in many cases of this complaint. Many of the pathogenetic effects of this drug likewise indicate it as a remedy of considerable value in Diabetes: there is a dry, itching skin; a yawning kind of sleeplessness; ill-humour; weakness of memory; continuous stinging pain in the liver; constipation, and a frequent desire to urinate, both by day and night, with general languor and weariness of the limbs.

LACTIC ACID. — Professors Cantani and Primavera, of Naples, report the most encouraging success from the use of two to four scruples of Lactic Acid, in six ounces of water, with each meal. The diet consists entirely of meat, including fish; half a drachm of alcohol to one ounce of water being allowed at dinner. Perseverance with the treatment, even for several months after the disappearance of sugar from the urine, is necessary.

LEDUM PALUSTRE. — Laurie and the *"North American Examiner"* refer to this drug as a remedy in Diabetes. Its pathogenesy relative to the leading characteristics runs as follows: — There is particular heat of the hands and feet; aching pains and chronic swelling of the joints; skin very dry, with itching herpes, boils, and carbuncles; sleeplessness, and restless tossing about in bed; anxiety, and general restlessness of mind; tubercles on the forehead, as in drunkards; constipation, and frequent and copious discharge of urine.

LEPTANDRA VIRGINICA. — This American preparation has done me good service in several cases of Diabetes Mellitus arising from, or coupled with, a congested condition of the liver. It acts upon the liver with energy, without active catharsis,

MAGNESIA CARBONICA. — Laurie, in one of his "Domestics," refers to this preparation as a Diabetic medicine. We have, as its pathogenesy, a relaxed condition of the body, loss of strength, and general debility; a dry, pricking, and itching condition of the skin; restless sleep, anxious dreams, ill-humour, and a desponding mood; itching of the hairy scalp, and a falling-off of the hair; violent thirst; dull pain, with a sensation of something hard in the liver; great heaviness in the abdomen; stools costive; copious pale or green urine, and a diminution of the sexual instinct.

MERCURIUS SOLUBILIS. — Hempel, Pulte, Laurie, Small, and Ruddock refer to Mercurius Solubilis as a remedy in Diabetes Mellitus. This medicine, as well as the Iodide of Potassium, may yield considerable benefit in these cases where a syphilitic taint in the constitution is suspected. On the urinary group the pathogenetic effects of Mercury are striking. We first notice enuresis. Mercury, if administered in large doses, causes an increased secretion of urine; and it not only causes an increased and almost irrepressible desire to urinate, but it occasions the deposition of sediment, which may yield very important therapeutic indications. According to the statement of our provers, the urine, under the influence of Mercury, deposits a whitish, flocculent sediment.

One record reads thus: —

"Shreds and flocks of whitish mucus are passed after micturition."

Another prover records this symptom: —

"The urine is at first clear, but afterwards looks whitish, as if mixed with chalk."

Another record: —

" The urine looks as" if stirred with flour, depositing a thick sediment."

These symptoms, coupled with the fact that Mercury causes the secretion of increased quantities of a watery urine, far surpassing in quantity the amount of beverage drank, might lead us to employ Mercury both in Diabetes Mellitus and in Albuminuria. It is, however, unfortunate, as I have already observed, that no chemical analysis was made of these sediments, as well as of many others; and that we are, therefore, left to guess whether the sediments were of a mucous, albuminous, or saccharine character.

NATRUM MURIATICUM (common salt).— In the *"Archiv. fur Anatome and Physiologie,"* Drs. Bock and Hoffman have stated, that the injection of a weak solution of common salt into the carotids or crural artery of a rabbit, produces Diabetes Mellitus. Firstly, polyuria takes place; then comes the sugar, which reaches a maximum quantity, and then gradually ceases. This is highly suggestive of Natrum Muriaticum as a Homoeopathic remedy.

The pathogenetic effects of Nat. Mur., as proved by Hahnemann and his immediate friends, mark it as a remedy in rheumatic, scrofulous, hysterical, and paralytic affections: the skin is dry, and itches all over the body; restless, yawning sleep; micturition every hour of the night; dejection of spirits; and hypochondriasis; palpitation of the heart; absence of mind; weak memory; frequent feeling of hunger; excessive appetite; constant thirst; aching, stitching pains in the liver; tension of the abdomen; frequent unsuccessful urging at stool; frequent micturition, both by day and night; discharge of mucus from the urethra; impotence.

NUX VOMICA.— The action of the Strychnos Nux Vomica on man, constitutes three separate degrees.

1. It acts as a tonic and diuretic, by promoting the appetite, and increasing the secretion of urine.

2. It promotes rigidity, and convulsive contraction of the muscles.

3. It causes tetanus, asphyxia, and death.

Nux Vomica affects, primarily, the spinal column, motor and sentient nerves. Nux Vom. also affects the brain. We infer this from the fact that it has caused stupor, vertigo, buzzing in the ears, sleeplessness, and turgescence of the capillaries of the face. Nux Vom., according to Flourens, acts on the cerebrum as well as the cerebellum; for both hemispheres of the brain have been found softened after death, particularly the latter. Nux Vom. also acts upon the medulla oblongata; from which we ought to anticipate brilliant results to follow the administration of Nux Vom. in cases of Diabetes Mellitus arising from disease of that portion of the nervous system. Nux Vomica can boast of as extensive a range of action upon the chylo-poietic viscera, as any other drug in the British Pharmacopoeia or Materia Medica. It successfully copes with the various derangements of taste, appetite, salivary secretions, dyspepsia, the liver, and bowels. It controls incontinence of urine, nocturnal enuresis, strangury, catarrh of the bladder; and, in view of the remarkable action which Nux V. has upon the functions of the liver, as marked by a throbbing, tensive pain and pressure in the liver, with occasional jaundice, and a copious pale-coloured urine, we should expect from Nux V. brilliant results in cases of Diabetes arising from a congested condition of the liver.

PLUMBUM METALLICUM, says Ruddock, promises to be a successful remedy in Diabetes Mellitus, as its action is specifically on the kidneys. The provings and toxicological effects of Plumbum, however, show that it diminishes the secretion of urine; it causes a perfect retention of urine; tenesmus at the neck of the bladder, with burning in the urethra; the urine looks saturated, brown, and mixed with blood; and, to my mind, is in more specific *rapport* with Ischuria and Haematuria than Diabetes.

PODOPHYLLUM PELTATUM— otherwise known as May-apple, Hog-apple, or Mandrake — has done me good service in several cases of Diabetes Mellitus connected with a congested condition of the liver, and a fagged brain, and, may be, an abnormal condition of the hepatic cells.

This medicine, of American birth, was first proved by Williamson, Jeanes, Ward, and Hussman, who recommend it in congestions of internal organs, more especially the liver and spleen; congestive headache; hypochondriasis; indigestion; headaches from disordered digestion; dysentery; prolapsus ani; haemorrhoids; dropsy, &c.; thus clearly showing its marked influence over a congestive condition of the chylopoietic viscera. Podophyllum rouses the liver to vigorous action; it determines the blood to the surface; it stimulates the kidneys, promotes expectoration, augments the glandular functions, and cleanses the intestinal canal of all irritating substances. Podophyllum may therefore prove a potent remedy in those cases of Diabetes, the chief cause of which may be traced to a congested condition and uniform enlargement of the liver, with an abnormal condition of the secreting cells, whereby the Grlucogene is imperfectly assimilated, and thereby passes from the system by the urine as saccharine matter. It were useless to administer this medicine in any other form than in its crude condition — either the matrix tincture or the 1st or 2ndx trituration.

CALCAREA SULPHURATA, vel HEPAR SULPH. — This preparation has been recommended for Diabetes; but I fear with but little benefit.

SALYCILIC ACID. — This preparation, in 10-grain doses, thrice a-day, is said to have reduced the sugar and amount of urine, and so far relieved all other symptoms as to enable the patient to partake of starchy substances.

STRYCHNINE, being so closely allied to Nux Yom. — being, in fact, its active alkaloid principle — offers the same pathogenetic, consequently, curative effects as Nux Vom.

SULPHUR. — Both Pulte and Laurie give Sulph. in their list of medicines as a remedy in Diabetes.

Generally, Sulphur is principally adapted to lymphatic temperaments, venous constitutions, with a tendency to haemorrhoids: there is general itching of the skin; despondency; pain, pressure, and contraction in the liver; constipation; piles; frequent micturition, which is copious both by day and night: the urine is clear.

STAPHYSAOEIA. Small refers to this medicine in Diabetes. On the urinary organs it produces a frequent desire to pass a large quantity of pale, watery urine, with sometimes a painful micturition.

TEREBINTHINE. — At length we hope a drug has been found that will cause sugar to appear in the urine. That drug is the Terebinthine.

According to the investigation of a German physician, Dr. Almen, he has succeeded in detecting sugar in the urine of patients that had been taking turpentine. By means of an alkaline solution of bismuth, it can be demonstrated, that the urine of patients taking an emulsion of turpentine becomes saccharine as soon as they have taken a quantity of emulsion equivalent to about 100 drops of the Oleum Terebinthine.

Dr. Burnett, of Birkenhead, in the case of a girl, aged twenty, after having treated her with China and Nitrate of Uranium with no benefit, found considerable improvement, in all the symptoms, to follow Terebinthine 3x.

URANIUM NITRATE. — Dr. McLaran records the following case of Diabetes cured by Uranium: — Bertie, aged three, of healthy parents, had been treated for dyspepsia and worms: was afterwards seen by Dr. McLaran, who suspected Diabetes. The urine had a saccharine odour, which was detected by Trommer's test. Nitrate of Uranium, 3x, was administered three times a-day for three weeks, when the urine was found normal, and the general health much improved.

VERATEUM ALBUM. — Small is the only authority known to me who refers to Verat. Al. as a remedy in Diabetes. Its efficacy is, however, doubtful.

Chapter Ten - Hydropathy As an Auxiliary in The Treatment of Diabetes

IT is a somewhat remarkable fact, that, up to the present time, scarcely any attention has been devoted to Hydropathy by the many eminent physicians who have made Diabetes Mellitus their *special* study, and who have contributed largely to the literature of the subject. Pavy, Harley, and Donkin make no reference whatever to this subject; and the only allusion to be found in Copland's colossal "Dictionary of Medicine" on the point is, that he recommends " the occasional use of vapour and alkaline baths, with woollen clothing worn next the skin." Much, however, I am fully persuaded, may be done with judiciously selected hydropathic appliances, both as curative and palliative agents, in the treatment of this hitherto-considered intractable complaint. One of the most common and prominent symptoms of Diabetes Mellitus is a dry, parched, scaly, and unperspirable condition of the skin. The seven million of pores which feed the surface of the cutaneous envelope are hermetically sealed. The vital functions of the skin, in relation to the animal economy, are not sufficiently understood, and far too much pooh-poohed and greatly underrated, because not properly studied and understood. The investigations, however, of modern physiologists, aided by powerful microscopic agency, have clearly revealed its truly marvellous organism, and demonstrated bow all-essential its sound and active vitality is to the due performance of the functions of healthy life; and also bow it is designed as a medium through which, in cases of disease, the internal organism can be safely reached and acted on.

The skin, in the popular acceptation of the term, is considered as only ONE single structure; but in reality, what, in ordinary language, is called the skin, is, to the anato-physiologist, known as the epidermis — the outer or scarf-skin — underneath which lies the "cutis vera," or true skin. Thus, properly speaking, the skin consists of two layers — the inner layer, and, immeasurably, the more sensitive and delicate, being known as the cutis vera, the derma, or true skin — and the outer layer, by which the cutis is protected, as the epidermis, or scarf-skin. Between these two layers, or strata, there is a soft, granular, or cellular substance called the rete mucosum, which contains a certain substance that gives the colour to the skin.

Some physiologists hold, that the matter which gives colour to the skin is situated in the rete mucosum; while others are of opinion that it lies in the inner or flocculent surface of the epidermis. According to Beddoes, chlorine gas will extract the colouring matter from the negro; and Fourcroy verified this experiment: but in a few days the black colour returned again with its former intensity.

"The skin," says Carpenter, "is concerned in two great classes of changes:

" 1. The excretion of various matters from its surface, and from the various glands in its substance.

" 2. The reception of impressions upon the nerves, with which it is so copiously supplied."

Thus the skin performs analogous functions to the lungs, in so far as it takes in and gives out similar matters, which are taken in and given out by the lungs; and for this reason it has been described as "the assistant apparatus of the lungs."

In health the skin is the seat of various secretions, which seek the surface of the body, to be eliminated, as excrementitious and deleterious matter, from the system. These secretions are collected in small glandular organs, which are seated just beneath the cutis, or true skin, and are diffused over the whole surface of the body to an extent that is truly marvellous. From these glandular organs, innumerable minute tubes, popularly called "the pores of the skin," convey the secretions through the epidermis, or outer scarf-skin, to be exuded in sensible or insensible perspiration. When Nature has destined these pores to perform so important a function and office, it can be readily understood how essential it is to health, that the normal action of the pores should not, in any way, be obstructed. This becomes still more apparent when we come to consider the very minute organism of the skin, and the wonderful system of pore-sewerage which Nature has provided for the healthy maintenance of human life. That able anatomist and dermatologist, Erasmus Wilson, says — "To arrive at something like an estimate of the value of the perspiratory system in relation to the rest of the organism, I counted the perspiratory pores on the palm of the hand, and found 3,528 in a square inch. Now each of these pores being an aperture of a little tube of about a quarter of an inch long, it follows that, in a square inch of skin on the palm of the hand, there exists a length of tube equal to 882 inches, or 73 1/2 feet. Surely such an amount of drainage as seventy-three feet in every square inch of skin, assuming this to be the average for the whole body, is something wonderful; and the thought naturally intrudes itself, What if this gigantic system of drainage were obstructed, or even partially so? Could we need a stronger argument for enforcing the absolute necessity of paying strict attention to the skin?

"To obtain an estimate of the length of the tube of the perspiratory system of the whole surface of the body, I think 2,800 might be taken as a fair average of the number of pores in a square inch, and 700, consequently, of the number of inches in length. Now, the number of square inches of surface in a man of ordinary height and bulk is 2,500; the number of pores therefore will amount to 7,000,000; and the number of inches of perspiratory tubing may be estimated at 1,750,000: that is, 145,833 feet; or 48,600 yards; or nearly 28 miles; " and which would extend from London to Windsor.

Now, the secretions of the human system are constantly going on, and, in a normal or healthy condition of the body, the portion assigned to be exhaled, or passed out by the skin, is carried off imperceptibly by the pores in the form of perspiration. The entire amount of fluid thus insensibly evaporated by the pores is estimated at eleven grains per minute; while the lungs, so sensibly in motion, and, apparently, more active, only evaporate about seven grains. Carpenter says, " There is reason to believe that at least 100 grains of azotised matter are excreted from the skin daily." Consequently, any cause which checks this excretory power of the skin must necessarily throw an additional and unnatural amount of labour on the other excretory organs of the system — viz., the lungs and kidneys — and thereby tend to produce a derangement of their functions, and cause disease. According to Dr. Thudichum, the secretion of the human skin may be divided into volatile and solid; the former consisting of —

1. Carbonic acid, water, and some volatile acid, not yet accurately determined.

2. Urea, chloride of sodium, fatty matter, earthy salts of some fatty solids, and small quantities of some other alkaline salts. Phosphates and sulphates, always present in any other secretion, have not, he says, been ever found in perspiration.

Thus, while the excretions of the skin are analogous, to some extent, to those of the lungs and kidneys, they are not entirely so. But its dignity as an excretory organ becomes more apparent from a careful study of the quantities of matter discharged by the several excreting organs of the body; for while the lungs, in twenty-four hours, discharge fifteen ounces of volatile matter, the skin discharges thirty ounces; so that two-thirds of all volatile excretions pass by the skin. An almost equal weight of water leaves the body through the kidneys, charged with matter peculiar to that secretion. We can thus understand how it is that the suppression of skin-action becomes a frequent source of disease. It is not, however, as an emunctory or purifier only that we must regard the skin; its influence and power have a far wider range of action in the maintenance of health. Besides comprehending a vast labyrinthian system of drainage tubes, which open on its surface by over seven millions of pores; besides, also, a wonderful and perpetual labour, by which the skin is drawing from the blood certain organic elements in the fluid state, and converting them into solid organic formations, which are known as cells and scales; these cells and scales being tesselated mosaic, with which the skin is furnished upon the surface so as to render it capable of existence in the external world; — besides this, and much more, the skin is converted into a kind of sponge, by the myriads of blood-vessels which enter into its structure — blood vessels so small as not to be seen by the naked eye; blood-vessels that, many times in an hour, bring the whole — aye, every drop — of the blood of the body to the surface; bring it, that it may furnish the materials for the microscopic pavement; that it may be purified by the abstraction of its unwholesome principles — its dross; that it may inhale the pure air of heaven without; — besides this, also, the skin near its surface is one vast network of nerves — nerves, mysterious organs, that belong, in their nature, to the unknown sources of the lightning, the electric currents of the vast universe. And besides these, again, there is every variety of animal tissue and contrivance by which all this wonderful apparatus is held together and maintained in the best state and position to ensure its safety and perfection. In truth, the contemplation of the structures and functions of the skin, when viewed with the eye of the mind, is almost overwhelming; and the words of the poet break upon our memory: —

> "In human works, though labour'd on with pain,
>   A thousand movements scarce one purpose gain;
>   In God's, one single can its end produce,
>   Yet serves to second, too, some other use."

One word more as to the importance of the skin in the animal economy, and that word a summary of its functions and principal vital attributes.

The SKIN is a sanitary commissioner, draining the system of its impurities.

The SKIN is an energetic labourer, in that perpetual interchange of elements which, in its essence, constitutes life.

The SKIN is a regulator of the density and fluidity of the blood.

The SKIN performs the office of a lung in supplying the blood with oxygen, and abstracting its carbon.

The SKIN changes the crude organic elements of the blood, so as to render them capable of nutrition.

The SKIN emulates the heart in giving speed to the general circulation of the blood.

The SKIN is the minister of the brain and spinal marrow, in its properties of sensation.

The SKIN feeds, as it were, nourishes, and keeps in the highest operative condition, that part of the nervous system which is confided to its care.

Viewing the SKIN in this way, and recognising its just claims to consideration as an important animal organ, we are led to the conclusion that the skin is a part of the "digestive system," like the liver and kidneys, by virtue of its emunctory and nutritive powers; it is an appendage of the heart, and a part of the system of the circulation of the blood; it is a surface lung, a breathing organ; and it partakes of man's intellectual nature by its close connection with, and dependence on, the brain. In the lower animals, the skin combines in itself alone, the FEELING, SEEING, SMELLING, HEAKING, and JUDGING ORGANS.

From this it will be clearly perceived how vitally essential a sound condition of the skin is to the enjoyment of good health. When its functions are impaired, or imperfectly performed, the whole body necessarily suffers. The heart, the lungs, the liver, the stomach, the bowels, the brain, and nerves, are imperfectly nourished, and their healthy vitality is more or less oppressed and weakened by the noxious matters with which the blood is loaded. Thus a heavy weight is placed on the very mainsprings of life; while it is only by restoring the healthy functions of the skin that this weight can be taken off.

We have further proof of the vast importance of healthy skin-action to life, in the fact that, if an animal be coated over with a varnish impervious to air, by which means the functions of the skin become impeded, and its organism, as it were, paralysed, death, in a few hours, would be the inevitable result. This has been demonstrated both on animals and man. Close the pores of his skin by a similar coating, and congestion of the internal organism would take place, followed, sooner or later, by death.

It is an irresistible conclusion, therefore, in which all eminent physiologists agree,, that whatever interferes with, or impedes perfect skin-action, must be more or less detrimental to health, and calculated, of necessity, to engender disease. When the functions of the skin are seriously interfered with, it usually happens that derangements,, more or less serious, either of the kidneys, lungs, or the liver occur. And just as that interference is permitted to continue — in proportion as it is perniciously prolonged — so will functional as well as organic derangements of the internal organism be intensified, and rendered still more organic and incurable.

Dr. Copland, in his edition of Richrand's "Physiology," refers to cases that came under his own observation, which remarkably illustrated the marvellous vital functions of the skin. The lungs, he says, " were partly destroyed from an imposthume, and the side of the chest was consequently contracted." Nevertheless, he found that the cutaneous functions increased, so as to supply the deficiency caused by impaired lung-action. All subsequent experience has tended to establish the potent agency of the skin, not only as an "assistant to the lungs," but also to the whole excretory organism; for it is a well-established fact, that there is an anatomical connection between the mucous membrane which lines our internal organism, and the external mucous membrane, or true skin, which covers the whole body. The general term, " mucous membrane," may be applied to that great system of membranous expansions which forms the external tegument, or skin — the lining of the internal cavities, whose walls are continuous with it; or mucous membrane proper — and the prolongation of this into the secreting organs, forming the tubes and follicles of the glands. Hence, in fact, the lungs are nothing but a bit of skin turned in, just as the internal surface of the lung would become skin if it were exposed externally. Unfortunately, however, medical practitioners have not heretofore properly understood the marvellous functions of the skin, and therefore did not seek to make available as sound physiology and pathology now dictates.

The skin was not regarded as supplying a medium through which deranged internal organism could be easily reached, and remedially acted on; but was rather viewed as a substance *"per se,"* liable to many diseased conditions, which medical art sought to cure either by experimental external revulsives — as ointments, lotions, blisters, issues, moxas, cupping, leeching, and other tormenting appliances, &c. — or by the administration of drugs to act through the digestive process. No organ, in fact, has been more misunderstood, neglected, and ill-used than the skin; and drug medication is still deplorably at fault as regards the possession of specifics, not only with respect to internal diseases, but those proper to the skin as well.

The revival of hydropathy, as practised by the Asclepiades of ancient Greece, and the resuscitation of the Tepidarium, Calidarium, and Frigidarium (Turkish), or Roman bath of ancient Rome, is fast becoming recognised as a most valuable hygienic means, not only as a preservator of health, but as a radical curative agent in a large number of diseases, many of which had hitherto baffled the efficacy of the most approved allopathic treatment.

It is by the proved amenability of the organism to the soothing, yet stimulating and nourishing influence of hot air, that the great remedial virtues of the Roman bath, judiciously administered, are brought into action, and are enabled to operate. This truth is now so well established, that it is already producing revolutionary changes of the greatest import in the present confused and contradictory theories of medical practice.

TURKISH BATH.— In Diabetes Mellitus, its value as an auxiliary and help-mate can scarcely be realised: it relieves all internal congestions; it abstracts from the blood all deleterious matter; it keeps up a normal action of the skin; it is a preservative of that balance of nutritive functions of the body which, in its essence, is health; it removes excessive fatigue, both mental and bodily; soothes the whole system, and gives the patient calm and refreshing sleep.

This bath should be taken three or four times a week. In some of my cases I have prescribed it to be taken daily, and have been much pleased with its beneficial effects.

VAPOUR BATH AND THE SPIRIT-LAMP BATH. — In the absence of the Turkish bath, which cannot at the present time be obtained in every town, village, or hamlet, we possess, in the vapour and spirit-lamp baths, admirable substitutes, which can be used at home and in our own bedroom. In past centuries, every known country, whether civilised or uncivilised, had its bagnio, or sweating house, however rude and primitive in its construction. The remains of these baths, which are in the shape of an oven, are still found in some remote parts of Ireland, Finland, and North America, even as far as the slopes of the Rocky Mountains; Japan, China, Egypt, Russia, and in the far-off Bokhara in Central Asia.

VAPOUR BATH— *Directions.*— The patient, being undressed, sits on a chair; a blanket is then put round the body, covering the whole person in the chair, leaving out the head only; two or three more blankets, rugs, or any other kind of thick coverlids of the same kind, are adjusted over the blanket in a similar way; taking care to close each separately well round the neck, and let them fall on the floor, so as to keep out the cold air, and keep in the hot steam. Then pour about a gallon of boiling water into an earthenware pan, or a wooden pail; put a brick, a piece of iron or coke, RED-HOT, in the water; place the vessel under the chair, closing the blankets well up all round the neck and floor, when perspiration will soon be produced. During the bath, some cold water should be given, by sips, to encourage perspiration; and the forehead may be sponged with cold water. After the patient has perspired freely for from fifteen to twenty minutes, all the clothes must he thrown off, and a cold dripping sheet or shallow bath given, followed by rapid friction all over the body with the Turkish or Baden-Baden towels, and particularly over" the region of the liver, and up and down the spine.

SPIRIT-LAMP— *Directions.* — This bath is a still more simple and convenient one, and, on the whole, more efficacious. It is given in the same way, and followed by the dripping sheet or shallow bath; only, instead of the boiling water, brick, iron, or coke, a lighted lamp, containing spirits of wine or methylated spirit (which is much cheaper, and quite as good), is placed under and in the centre of the chair. The process takes about the same time as the vapour bath, and is of great help in the treatment of dropsy, chronic diseases of the liver, various skin affections, and in Diabetes Mellitus.

LIVER COMPRESS. — I have frequently recommended the liver compress in cases of Diabetes Mellitus, when I had reason to suspect that organ to be at fault. If worn continuously for a week or ten days, it generally brings out a thick crop of pustules, with marked relief to anything like a feeling of congestion in that organ. It removes congestion, and rouses the organ to increased action; which is clearly indicated by an increased flow of bile, and a more active condition of the bowels.

WET BODY-PACK. — Next in importance and efficacy to the Turkish and vapour baths, is the wet pack. — Directions, — Spread a mackintosh sheet, or thick quilt, on a mattress, and over that one or two dry blankets; then take a thick cotton or linen sheet, dip it in cold water, and wring the water out as much as possible. This is more effectually done by two persons, by twisting the sheet — first doubled up — in a reversed direction. It is now shook out and laid evenly on the mattress. The patient, being undressed, lies down upon the back on the wet sheet, holding up the arms while one side of it is thrown over the body and tucked in; then the patient puts the arms down by the side of the body, and the other part of the wet sheet is thrown over all, and tightly tucked in; the blanket and mackintosh are then brought over, on each side, in a similar manner; a bed, or plenty of blankets or clothes, is next put on the patient, so as to keep the body warm.

1. It is very important, in packing, that the sheet be well wrung out.

2. It is also important that the patient be tightly packed in the sheet and blankets, particularly round the neck and feet, with the bed or plenty of clothes on. After being in the pack for one hour, or a little longer, the patient should take a cold dripping sheet, or shallow bath; after which a dry sheet. If delicate, use rubbing sheet at 70 degrees, and stand on a warm pad, or in hot water. Dress quickly, and then take moderate exercise.

Chapter Eleven - Dietetic Treatment of Diabetes Mellitus

THE object to be attained in the treatment of Diabetes (says Pavy), is to control the elimination of sugar; and according to the extent that this can be effected, the symptoms of the disease are subdued.

There are two plans of treatment in vogue, which, as" a rule, require to be put into practice together, namely —

1. Medicinal agents.

2. Dietetic agents.

With the first we aim at removing the pathological phenomena of the complaint — in fact, its cause, — when nature resumes her normal functions.

With the second we aim at avoiding feeding the disease, by selecting a diet devoid of saccharine matter.

I have already fully discussed the therapeutic and hydropathic agents as being applicable to the various causes of Diabetes. All that now remains is to refer to its dietetics, and mineral waters adapted to the complaint.

There are, however, some cases met with in which the disease has been removed by purely medicinal treatment. Four such cases have occurred in my own practice. It is, however, in the generality of cases. very essential that patients should conform to a particular code of dietetic rules, &c.

Prout expressed an opinion, that the first and chief point to be attended to in the treatment of Diabetes is diet. This, on the whole, is fully endorsed by most practitioners who have given special attention to this class of diseases.

The "Rationale" of this is very clear. Let us, by way of illustration, observe, that with a healthy person, when saccharine and farinaceous materials are ingested, as in partaking of bread, and many other vegetable articles of food, they are lost sight of in the system, because there exists an aptitude for assimilation, whereby they are rendered available for the requirements of life. Their physiological destination being fulfilled, their elements, it is presumed, escape chiefly in the form of carbonic acid and water from the body. With a Diabetic patient, however, similar food, instead of being appropriated to the nourishment of the body, is allowed to pass through the system unemployed. A piece of bread, for instance, being eaten, the starchy matter which the bread contains is converted into sugar by the ptyalin and pancreatin: but the transformation proceeds no further. There exists an incapacity, from some cause or other, in the sugar-manufacturing department of the liver, for carrying on the process of normal assimilation, and, as a consequence, the sugar so formed gets into the circulation, and from thence into the kidneys, by which organs it is discharged unchanged, and its passage through the system producing the train of abnormal phenomena which so prominently characterise the disease. The chief object, therefore, which the physician has in view in the treatment of Diabetes, is to place the constitution of the patient in as favourable a position, approaching the standard of health, as possible.

There are few diseases which present to the practitioner so clear an indication of what is to be done; and there are few diseases the management of which is so open to rational principles as Diabetes. An element of food, from some want of capacity in properly disposing of it, makes its appearance, as a foreign body, in the circulation, and gives to its contents an unnatural condition, which is detected in the renal secretion by the most simple chemical manipulation. If we consider for a moment the immense quantity of sugar which is sometimes voided by a Diabetic patient, evidence of which is presented both in the blood and other secretions, we cannot be surprised that a very serious deviation from the standard of health prevails.

Prout gives an instance of a patient who passed, under a mixed diet, twenty-one pints of urine, containing 47.05 grains of sugar to the fluid ounce, in twenty-four hours: rather more than 19,000 grains, or upwards of 2 ¾ lbs. of sugar, must have therefore traversed the circulation during that brief period.

Now, to reduce this abnormal condition of urine to the nearest approach to a healthy standard, is the chief point to be aimed at in treatment; and to obtain this object, a Diabetic should exclude all saccharine and farinaceous materials from his diet. This, to be strictly carried out, involves an abstinence from almost all the ordinary kinds of vegetable food. In carrying out, however, the exclusion of all the starch and sugar from the food, it is not necessary that complete restriction to animal food should be enforced, as there are many vegetable substances that may be allowed, and sufficient to admit of fair variation at meals. In lieu of bread, which contains about 70.5 per cent, of starch and sugar, and which must be strictly prohibited, there is now being regularly manufactured, for the special use of Diabetics, three kinds of food — the gluten, bran, and almond BREAD; upon each of which a few remarks are called for.

1. GLUTEN BREAD, which is a valuable nitrogenous, proteinaceous, or albuminous product of wheat, varying in amount from 11 to 15 per cent. It appears also that the quantity of gluten increases with the coarseness of the flour; and so also does the amount of mineral matter, of which phosphoric acid is the chief constituent. Wheat varies a good deal in composition according to season, climate, and soil; but as a rule, the cereals of southern climates and warm seasons are richer in gluten, and harder of texture, than that of cold climes. The nutritive value of gluten was discovered by Beccaria, more than a century ago, by the following process: — A given weight of flour — say 500 grains is made into rather stiff dough, and is carefully washed by tender manipulation under a small stream of water. The gluten remains, and when it is baked, it expands into a clean-looking ball, which should weigh, when thoroughly dried, about 54 grains. Bad flour makes a thin ropy-looking gluten, which is very difficult to deal with, and which has a dirty-brown colour when baked.

The manufacture of gluten bread was first undertaken at the suggestion of Dr. Bouchardat of Paris, who has published an able thesis on Diabetes Mellitus, wherein he suggests the use of gluten bread, and quotes cases showing the advantage of its employment. It is prepared in Toulouse and Paris, and imported into this country in the form of slices and rolls. It may be procured in London at Van Abbot's Dietetic Depot, 5, Princes Street, Cavendish Square. Gluten flour is also to be obtained at the same establishment, which may be applied to a variety of culinary purposes in the place of ordinary flour. Mr. Bonthron, of 106, Regent Street, London, has succeeded in manufacturing some gluten biscuits and bread, which are considered more palatable than those of Yan Abbot's. They eat short and crisp, and are readily reducible in the mouth.

2. BRAN BREAD. — Chemically, bran contains a good deal of nitrogenous matter; is rich in fat and saline substances. According to M. Mege Mourics, bran contains a portion of very soluble nitrogenous matter — CEREALINE, which is of the nature of DIASTASE — and has the property of dissolving

starch. The late Dr. Prout was about the first to recommend bran as a substitute for bread in Diabetes — consisting of a compound of bran, eggs, and milk. The late Dr. Camplin, who had been a sufferer from Diabetes for many years, was able to keep the enemy at bay, and prolong life, by the use of this bread, and suggested some improvement in its mode of manufacture, by proposing a combination of bran and gluten.

Mr. Blatchley, of 362 Oxford Street, who for some years worked under Dr. Camplin's instructions, now prepares the bran bread according to his recommendation; and is now known as Blatchley's Bran Gluten Biscuits, being made from French gluten and prepared bran. Those who desire to make their own bran-gluten bread, can procure the flour, which is of excellent quality, from Messrs. Chapman and Co., St. James' Mills, Hatcham. The following is an excellent recipe for its preparation, as suggested by Pavy: —

Take 4oz. of prepared bran-flour, 1 drachm of bicarbonate of soda, 5 eggs, and about a quarter of a pint of warm milk. First mix the bicarbonate of soda with the bran-flour, then beat up 2oz. of butter in a hot basin, and shake into it the mixture of bran-flour and bicarbonate of soda, beating with a spoon all the while. Next beat up the five eggs in a separate basin before the fire till milk-warm, and stir them gradually into the mixture of bran-flour, soda, and butter. Beat up all well together for at least ten minutes, adding gradually the warm milk. Place in well-buttered tins, or patty-pans, and bake in a brisk oven for about ten minutes. The cakes are done when they will turn out of the tins quite easily. The above quantities will make about five cakes, of the size of ordinary buns. The cakes, if desired, may be cut into slices, toasted and buttered. Instead of all bran-flour, equal parts, or other proportions of bran and almond flour, may be used. The cakes, in the opinion of many, are thus rendered more palatable. The almond flour seems to soften and neutralise the taste of the bran, whilst the bran reduces the richness of the almond flour.

3. ALMOND BREAD. — This kind of Diabetic food was first suggested by Dr. Pavy. " Looking," he says, " at the drawbacks that existed with regard to the starchy grains, I turned my attention to products of the vegetable kingdom from which starch is absent. The almond is of this kind, and forms an edible and nourishing article. The hemp-seed also pretty closely resembles the almond in its chemical composition, and is to be purchased at considerably less cost; but there are difficulties in the way of separating the husk from the kernel, which deprive it of equal adaptability for the purpose of food."

The oily character of the almond renders it a very desirable article of food for the Diabetic. There is a want of power in the disease to turn to account one form of heat-producing food — namely, the saccharine and FARINACEOUS; whilst with the other, the oleaginous, there exists no difficulty. Theoretically, the Diabetic should be supplied pretty largely with fat; and, practically, it is found that its effect is highly beneficial.

Analysed by M. Boullay, they were found to contain —

A bland fixed oil	54 per cent.
Emulsine, a nitrogenised sub.stance	24 "
Sugar, in a liquid form	6 "
Gumwater	3 "
Woody fibre	4.0 "
Seed-coats	5 "
Which contain a little tannin	

Dr. Pereira, in his work on "Food and Diet," 1843, says, "Sweet almonds are nutritive and emollient, but, on account of their fixed oil, difficult of digestion, at least when taken in large quantities, or by persons whose digestive powers are weak." This also applies to the hazel-nut, filbert, walnut, Brazil nut, cocoa-nut, and, in fact, to all the oily seeds. Now the reason of their difficult digestibility is soon explained, and the difficulty at the same time easily overcome. In the process of digestion, the general opinion is, that all kinds of food are digested in the stomach alone by means of the gastric juice. This, however, is not so. Nitrogenous, proteinaceous, and albuminous substances, constituting as they do the leading articles of diet, are chiefly digested by the gastric juice and the intestinal mucus; but starchy substances and cellulose require the ptyalin of the saliva, and the pancreatin of the pancreatic fluid, as also the animal diastase of intestinal mucus, for that purpose; while fatty and oily matters are digested by the emulsifying action of the pancreatic fluid, and, may be, the bile; and by being thus broken up into extreme minute globules, they are freely admitted into the lacteal vessels. The more intimately the gastric juice can be incorporated with the constituent particles of the food, the more favourable will the circumstances be for the accomplishment of digestion. Now the difficult digestibility of the almond arises from the disadvantageous position under which it is placed, by virtue of its physical state, for being acted upon by the gastric fluid in the stomach. If we reduce it, however, to a fine powder before it enters the stomach, the process of digestion is not interfered with, and the almond becomes a most useful and nourishing food for Diabetic invalids. It is also a remarkable fact that oleaginous matters often agree better with Diabetics than other kinds of food; and that it has a tendency to increase the flow of saliva, consequently diminishes that urgent thirst which forms one of the most prominent symptoms of the complaint; and that it also gives a sensation of satisfaction and support to the stomach which other food frequently fails to do.

Mr. Blatchley, who supplies the bran-gluten biscuits, supplies also the almond biscuits, in an elegant-looking and palatable form.

In carrying out the dietery scheme required for excluding the ingestion of starchy and saccharine principles, I shall annex here two tabular forms — one containing articles of diet which should not be taken, the other containing articles of diet which may be taken.

Articles of Diet to Be Avoided.

1. Sugar. — Foremost among these is undoubtedly sugar, which should be strenuously avoided in any and every form.

2. Cereals. — Wheaten bread, and such-like food, whether derived from barley, oats, rye, Indian corn, millet, and Guinea corn. Preparations made from wheat: macaroni, vermicelli, Italian paste, and semolina; all of which abound more or less in sugar and starch.

3. Farinaceous Foods. — Arrowroot, sago, tapioca, and the various so-called farinaceous foods of infants.

4. Succulent Vegetable Foods. — The potato, turnips, parsnips, carrots, beetroot, and onions; the stem of leeks, asparagus, and the white heart of cabbages, secale, and cauliflower; all of which contain saccharine and starchy matter.

5. Leguminous Seeds, or Pulses. — Peas, broad-beans, French beans, or haricot, and lentil; which, like the cereals, contain a large amount of starch.

6. Ripe Fruits and Dry Fruits. — As apples, pears, peaches, pine-apples, and chestnuts; all of which abound in sugar and starch; also dried fruits, as dates, figs, grapes, raisins, and currants, which contain much sugar.

7. Drinks. —All malt liquors, as stout, porter, cooper, old and mild ale, cider, or perry; all sweet wines, sparkling wines, fruity port wines, liqueurs, and fresh milk.

8. Animal Food. — Ham, bacon, liver, or smoked, salted, dried, or cured meat.

Articles of Diet Which May Be Taken.

1. Almond, bran, or gluten, as prepared by the manufacturers, to act as a substitute for bread.

2. Animal Food. — As beef, mutton, venison, lamb, or veal, roasted, boiled, or grilled: poultry; any kind of game; and kind of fish, fresh, salted, or cured.

3. Soups, beef-tea, chicken or mutton-broth, thickened with gluten or almond flour; not, however, with any of the cereals, or their preparations.

4. Vegetables. — As spinach, tops of asparagus, turnip tops, artichokes, Brussels sprouts, and the green part of cabbages.

5. Salads. — Such as cress, mustard, endive, dandelion, the green portion of lettuce and watercress, with salad oil, vinegar, and a hard-boiled

6. Fresh vegetable gluten; that is, dough with the starch washed out, may be made into an agreeable little dish, with grated Parmesan or Gruyere cheese, and a little butter and an anchovy.

7. Home-made pickles may be taken in moderation, as they often act as a pick-up to an indifferent appetite.

8. Cream and butter may be used in making sauces, with some gluten or almond flour, or the yolk of an egg, to thicken.

9. Stimulating Beverages. — A selection may be made from the following white wines: — Dry sherries, Amontillado, Manzanilla, Montilla, Vinode-pasto, Chables, or Hock. Red Wines: a sound claret. Burgundy, or a Carlowitz. Those, however, who prefer it, may take, instead, a little good brandy, or very old whisky, with soda water. Seltzer water, Apollinaris water, or the Vichy or Freidrichshall water.

10. Morning and Evening Meal. — Cocoa, prepared from the nibs, and free from all fat and sugar; coffee or tea without sugar.

M. Bouchardat, Professor of Hygiene in the University of Paris, who has carefully studied the subject of Diabetes Mellitus, and the originator of gluten as a substitute for bread, gives us the following menu; which, as Dr. Chambers says, " has not been improved upon by subsequent writers on the subject:" —

INJURIOUS. — Sugar, bread of any kind, or pastry, rice, maize, and other starchy grains, potatoes, arrowroot, and tapioca, among root-products; sago, among piths; among manufactured starches — macaroni, vermicelli, and semolina; of vegetable seeds — peas and beans of all sorts, and chestnuts; radishes, turnips, beetroot, and carrots; beer, cider, sweet and sparkling wines, lemonades, and such-like sweetened acid drinks.

PERMISSIBLE.— Meat of all kinds, brown or white, boiled, roast, or grilled, and seasoned with any sauce pleasing to the palate, provided there be no SUGAR or FLOUR in it; all sorts of fish, shell-fish, and lobsters; eggs, cream, and cheese; spinach, endive, lettuce, sorrel, asparagus, hop-tops, artichokes, French beans, Brussels sprouts, cabbage (the last very good with pickled pork or bacon).

Salads of cress, endive, American cress, corn-salad, dandelion, lettuce, with a full allowance of oil and hard-boiled eggs. Fresh vegetable gluten — i. e., dough with the starch washed out — may be made into an agreeable dish, with grated Parmesan or Gruyere cheese and butter. Anchovy and Ravigote butter.

For dessert, olives: on high-days and holidays, when the patient has begun to improve, some fresh summer fruit — of course, without sugar. The wearing hunger may be much appeased by chewing the cocoa-beans.

For drink, a bottle and a-half of good claret or Burgundy may be taken in the day. Those who prefer it, may take, instead, brandy and soda-water: one part of the former to nine of the latter. Fresh beef tea is a capital quencher of thirst. Coffee, with cream.

It will here be observed, that the most serious privation a Diabetic is subject to, is the deprivation of bread. It is a most painful task imposed upon the physician to do so; but the eminently injurious properties of its starchy components leaves him no other alternative. Dr. Chambers expresses an opinion that it is not wise to enforce a diet which is really intolerable to the patient. He would conciliate the stomach, appetite, and fancy into taking the greatest amount of animal food and oleaginous matter possible; and if the patient ate the heartier for having a biscuit, or a crust, or a glass of porter, or even the forbidden fruit in the form of a vegetable with his meals, he would deem it better to give him his way than to tempt him to break through the rules altogether by playing the truant. It were better, however, to resist the temptation and craving with stoical bravery; and we should fortify the resolve to save life at all costs of self-denial. The dietetic treatment introduced by Dr. Eollo consists in restricting the patient to a purely animal food (all vegetable matter being excluded), comprising meat — fat beef, mutton, pork, and game — fish, oysters, light-boiled eggs, and a mixture of milk, and beef or mutton decoction, and water for drink. The meat to be cooked, but no seasonings allowed except a little salt. Dr. Rollo strictly enjoined the importance of restricting the animal food taken to a certain limited quantity.

Chapter Twelve - Hygienic Treatment

IN addition to a regular course of Turkish baths, and other hydropathic appliances, active muscular exercise daily, in the open air, may be considered as a valuable addenda to our code of treatment of Diabetes Mellitus.

M. Bouchardat, the Professor of Hygiene to the Faculty of Medicine in Paris, whose valuable contributions to this subject deserve our gratitude and highest encomiums, has more recently urged that equal attention should be paid to other points of an hygienic nature. He maintains that considerable benefit is derived from active muscular exercise, carried out in the open air every day; and he is in the habit of recommending his patients to go through a daily course of exercise at a gymnasium, or to subject themselves to some kind of work or exercise sufficiently active to throw them into a good perspiration. By this, he is of opinion, that a return of power of appropriating the starchy and saccharine elements of food is promoted. Special care should, at the same time, be taken to keep the skin warm and dry; that the mind should be kept calm and contented — free from mental work, care, sorrow, or anxiety; so that we may be able to exclaim, with Juvenal —

"Mens Sana in corpore sano."

Dr. Kulz, of Marburg, has observed eight cases of Diabetes Mellitus in which active exercise was of decided value; but such exercise must consist in vigorous movement in the open air; simple in-door gymnastics are scarcely of the slightest use. In his experience, the best results are obtained by mountain-climbing; and, provided the patients are fond of such exercise, and can support the necessary exertion, he strongly recommends this treatment in lieu of drugs, provided that careful preliminary experiments have shown that exercise diminishes the excretion of sugar in the particular cases.

"In addition to strict diet and regimen," says Copland, "a patient so afflicted should remove to a dry and warm situation, should constantly wear woollen next his skin, and keep up a free cutaneous discharge by suitable exercise."

"While patients are under treatment," says Donkin, "I am in the habit of prescribing out-door exercise, especially walking, or working in the garden. The main object of such prescriptions is to call into play a more active condition of the skin." This, however, is more effectually done by means of the Turkish and other sweating-baths, followed by active walking exercise.

Chapter Thirteen - Mineral Waters: Their Uses as Beverages and Medicinal Agents in Diabetes Mellitus

ONE of the most distressing symptoms which affects the Diabetic, is a constant and unquenchable thirst, an inordinate flow of urine, a torpid condition of the bowels, and a congested condition of the liver.

Now to relieve and assuage those terrible pangs of thirst, to replace the constant outpouring of fluid from the blood, and to rouse the dormant functions of the alimentary canal and liver, is one of the most important points which occupies the mind of the physician, and which, from day to day, taxes his inventive powers to suggest some more agreeable and palatable beverage than plain water.

It is true that the water which comes from the rippling mountain-stream, the village spring, the gladsome singing rill of woodland mossy slopes, the canopy of heaven, and that grand terrestrial filter the strata of the earth, gladdens the heart, soothes the mind, and quenches the thirst for a time; But the Diabetic, like other invalids, gets tired of its sameness, and craves for some more genial and palatable beverage.

For this purpose, we have admirable and inviting substitutes in soda-water, Seltzer water, and the gaseous Apollinaris water, as quenchers of thirst; and for the latter, the saline waters of Carlsbad; the alkaline waters of the renowned Vichy and Vals, and the bitter waters of Freidrichshall and Kissingen.

The soda-water, the Seltzer water, and the Apollinaris water, may be taken as ordinary beverages, either alone or with a little of the best French brandy; or, better still, some good old Scotch whisky.

After the first intensity of the disease has been subdued, we may then select one of the alkaline mineral waters. The Vals is the strongest of this class: and of the various springs at Vals, the Magdalene yields the strongest water. The Vichy waters come next in strength: they are situated in central France, and are, perhaps, the most celebrated in the whole world. The locality of Vichy is charming; the climate is mild, and hot in summer. They are celebrated in kidney disease, gout, liver derangement, and Diabetes, dyspepsia, and congestion of the spleen. The Vichy water holds in solution carbonic acid, bicarbonate of soda, bicarbonate of potash, bicarbonate of magnesia, strontia, lime, protoxide of iron, protoxide of manganese, sulphate of soda, phosphate of soda, arsenate of soda, borate of soda, chloride of sodium, silica, and bituminous organic matter. The Vichy water may sometimes be taken with meals, either alone or mixed with a sound claret or Burgundy, a Carlowitz, or a good old whisky.

The Freidrichshall is a bitter saline, not unlike the Pullna: it has laxative properties, and acts energetically on the liver, stomach, urinary organs, and pancreas.

Kissingen. — These celebrated waters rest on three springs, the most important of which is that known as the Ragoczy. In chronic congestion of the principal organs of the abdomen, the stomach, liver, spleen, pancreas, and kidneys, mesenteric and haeraorroidal vessels, the Ragoczy waters have acquired great reputation.

Those who are unable to procure these waters, or visit the spas of France and Germany, may find substitutes equally as potent in the saline waters of Cheltenham, Leamington, Stratford (in Essex), Kingswood (in Gloucestershire), and lastly — though not the least of them — the celebrated saline, sulphur, and cuprosaline and chalybeate waters of Llandrindod, situated amongst the Radnorshire mountains.

Llandrindod has long been the principal spa in Wales. The Mid-Wales train sets you down in the middle of an open, airy plain, at the foot of which rolls down the noble Eithon, celebrated for its salmon trout and graylings. Llandrindod, after being considered dreary, remote, and vacant of elegant accommodation after the middle of the last century, attracted for a time by its gambling, which gave it an unenviable reputation. It has, till very recently, been chiefly visited by the natives of the principality; but since the opening of the railway, visitors flock from other and more remote parts of England. There has been much facetiousness about the arrangements of the old hotel, which are still in force. There are two scales of charges, and two tables. The guests are divided into the Houses of Lords and Commons; and it is not considered correct for members of the UPPER to associate with members of the Lower House. The old saline and sulphur springs are situated some eight or nine minutes' walk from the railway-station, in a grove of fine, old, stately trees; where, also, are the Houses of Lords and Commons. Here is the principal pump-room, where the visitors assemble in the morning to drink the waters.

In 1755, Dr. Wessel Linden, a German physician, introduced the Radnorshire wells to the world by writing an elaborate work on their analysis and medicinal properties, a copy of which I possess. " The medicinal mineral waters," says the Doctor, "have ushered themselves into vogue by their own merit. No scribbling has ever been attempted in their favour, which I am well assured would never have availed there; for nothing but the extraordinary merits of their mineral contents could ever have rendered the place, from the condition it was in, a fit reception for the ' genteelest' company. Their good effects are so conspicuous, that they give way to none in Europe. I beg pardon for the boldness of this expression: but I beseech my readers to weigh it coolly, and to point out a water in EUROPE that can challenge the pre-eminence; I will then willingly give up my assertion. But I declare I have seen and made trial of several medicinal mineral waters, in divers parts of Europe, and have read of many more that have been tried by more able hands; but as yet I have not met with any, of the same kind, that surpass these at Llan-drindod."

Dr. Clermont, in 1720, says, in writing on these waters, that they were better for healing diseases than as drinking-water. For drinking, he preferred the Welsh ales. And

Drayton, in 1613, in alluding to some of the popular beliefs, relative to the efficacy of the waters, says,

"And on the Cambrian side,
Those strange and wondrous springs,
Our beasts that seldom drink."

SUB-NITRATE OF BISMUTH—*New Test for Diabetic Urine.* — To the suspected urine, add a solution of "one part of carbonate of soda in three parts of water," and boil the mixture with 15 or 30 grains of Sub-nitrate of Bismuth. When the fluid contains any GLUCOGENE, a black deposit is almost immediately formed; no change whatever occurring when no Diabetic sugar is present. This TEST is therefore perfectly distinct and characteristic.

www.ingramcontent.com/pod-product-compliance
Lightning Source LLC
Chambersburg PA
CBHW022124280326
41933CB00007B/531